Providence

Finding trust in God when He seems absent

JEFFRY L. PARKER

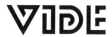

Vide Press
6200 Second Street
Washington D.C. 20011
www.VidePress.com

ISBN 978-1-7351814-2-4

Printed in the United States of America

Inscription

This book is inscribed to my loving, steadfast, and beautiful wife, my helpmate, without whom life would be incredibly dull, unexciting, and definitely less joyful.

Before You Buy

What this book is:

This book is a personal testimony about living out my faith during crises and how God provided for me and my family throughout all of my circumstances.

What this book is not:

I am not providing medical advice or a medical game plan. I am not qualified to do so. There are professionals who are. Please use their services to create the best game plan for you.

If you or your loved one is facing a difficult diagnosis, I do share what my wife and I went through and how we actively attacked my cancer in this book. Please know we shared our cancer battle plan with our medical staff and kept them informed every step of the way.

What would I advise:

When asked, the advice I give anyone facing a difficult diagnosis is to:

1. Take your case directly to the Great Physician, Jesus Christ, through prayer.
2. Learn everything you can about your illness and all available treatments.
3. Set realistic health goals—determine the best possible outcome and then work toward that goal.
4. Create a health plan—it's not a plan unless it's written down. Write the plan, and then share it with your health professionals. Keep it realistic.
5. Make informed decisions with your doctors. It's your decision to make—remember that.
6. Be honest with yourself and with your physicians at all times. Do not lie, no matter how embarrassing it may be to share the truth.
7. Be thankful, generous, and loving with your nurses. They take care of you.
8. Ask for prayer—get as many people praying for you as you can.
9. Do not give up! Keep fighting, keep praying, and keep hoping.

Acknowledgments

Thank you to Judy Post and Pastor Bill Van Loan for their invaluable assistance and insights as they reviewed and edited the manuscript. All our love!

Permissions

Table of Contents

Introduction

Jehovah Jireh—The Lord Will Provide

This true story has been waiting to be told in full for over a decade. I have shared parts of this story over the years in many different ways, but never have I told it in its entirety.

Everything I share in this book happened and is as I remember it. Any error is mine. The story is not just about me. Many other lives intersect in this story—my wife, my parents, my doctors, my nurses, my friends, and my extended family are all a part of this story. I have changed names where necessary.

There is one name I have not changed: the name who is the true author and the true subject of this story, my Lord and Savior Jesus Christ.

Prologue

I awakened slowly. I was flat on my back and unmoving, lying in a postoperative ward bed. The anesthesia had worn off just enough that I was beginning to become aware of my surroundings. Mentally, I was groggy and my eyelids felt anchored down, as if they were glued shut. The effort to open them was too much in my drugged state, so I kept them closed for now. The soft light of the post-op ward leaked through, assuring me I was awake.

This was my second surgery, and the growing familiar feeling of coming out of anesthesia was comforting, as if I had awakened out of a deep dream-filled yet restful sleep—a sleep so deep, it was slightly disorienting at first. I started to stretch my body when I realized I could not breathe.

My chest felt heavy, as if someone were sitting on it, compressing my lungs. I could not inhale or exhale. My stretch was short lived as the drugs were keeping me relatively immobile. As the reality of my inability to breathe hit me, my consciousness raced upward in a panic. My face and nose began to burn as the oxygen deprivation hit. My heart thudded in my chest, pumping blood and badly needed oxygen into my brain.

I flexed my fingers in a panic. I could hear someone in the room with me, and I needed to get their attention. Forcing my hands to move, I gripped the sides of the bed as tightly as I could. In my weakened state, I clenched my stomach muscles as much as I could, trying to force my lungs to function. The pain was enormous even through the pain medications. My abdominal muscles had been severed through only a few weeks before, and while healing had began, the muscles struggled to cooperate. I clenched through the pain, trying to force my lungs to do something, anything. My diaphragm spasmed slightly and pushed on my lungs, and water began to seep out of my nose and my mouth.

It was then I realized a horrifying fact: I was drowning, drowning in the middle of post-op.

Chapter 1

Where do I begin? How do I start this story? Do I start with nearly drowning in post-op? Do I start with the doctor giving me the cancer diagnosis? Do I start with my earliest memories of Christ? Where I start this story has been a struggle and one of the main reasons it has taken me so long to tell it. I suppose the best way to begin is to tell about my upbringing and background as a level set for the challenges that came into my life and are the core of the story.

My name is Jeff, and I was born and raised in northern Indiana. I grew up in the 1970s, which was a radically different time from today—not a better or a worse time, but just very different. Back in the 1970s, we had one or maybe two phones in the house, none of them cellular, and their mobile range was determined by the length of the cord attached to the handset. We had two phones. One phone was mounted on the kitchen wall, and the other sat on the bedside table in my parents' room.

Our TV had maybe three or four channels, sometimes five or six if the weather cooperated. The days we could pick up a channel from Lima, Ohio, were miracles. Top 40 radio stations were cool, and if we wanted, we could make our own playlists. We had to make mixtapes, recording songs off the radio and then compiling the songs together on cassettes ourselves. And, frankly, I did not wear a seatbelt riding in my parents' car or my grandfather's truck until

I was nearly eight years old. I had no clue what an infant car seat was, nor would I until the late 1980s.

In the '70s, the jobs in Indiana were limited to factory work, farming, insurance, retail, or military service. After my father left the military, he eventually took a job driving a long-haul truck all over the country. The job paid well, but it meant he was out of the house almost all of the time. He was home maybe two days out of every thirty. My mom worked a couple of different jobs until she landed the coveted school secretary job at a local elementary school. My school had a total of 97 students enrolled when I was in the sixth and final grade there. The school was blessed with tremendously dedicated teachers who cared deeply for their students.

With two parents working, my older brother and I spent a good amount of time alone or with our maternal grandparents, which was then, and is to this day, a true blessing. Our grandparents lived through the Great Depression and World War Two. At the time I did not realize it, but the Great Depression had left an indelible mark on them both. Grandma saved food—hoarded it, really. Lunches at her house were always smorgasbords. At lunch, we could be served pancakes, chicken, roast beef, Jell-O with fruit in it (a standard side dish), peas, carrots, and three different kinds of desserts on the table. All at one time! Lunch depended on the leftovers she had from the past week. I never left her house without feeling extremely full.

While Grandma taught us to waste nothing, from my grandfather I learned about having a strong work ethic, saving money, looking out for the "other guy," and loving our country. A clear lesson my grandfather always shared with me, in his own way, was about providing value. To put it simply, if someone hires me for a $5.00-an-hour job, the boss should expect me to give them $7.00 an hour worth of work. And if the employer takes advantage or does not appreciate the work or if it's just not a good fit, then don't complain; just thank them and move on. I work to adhere to this and many other valuable lessons, and I have passed them on to my family. The lessons I learned from my grandparents are extensive, and I am grateful for their willingness to share their lives with me. I once asked my grandfather what the Great Depression was like, and he just shrugged his shoulders and told me, "You worked harder and made less."

My maternal grandparents' lasting legacy, though—the one I am most thankful for—is their faith. They lived their faith like most people breathe, without conscious thought. Their faith was ever-present and it informed everything they did. I am not sure, but I do not believe it was a conscious or intentional process for them. It just was. I have to work at it. For them, their faith happened naturally.

They followed Christ seemingly without thinking about it. They were faithful, trusting Him as if He had proven Himself to them so thoroughly that there was no doubt, like He was with them every waking moment. It is their lives, walked in faith, that stand out in my mind and how their faith passed to my mom, to my brother, and then to me. I believe I was about five years old when I realized who Christ was and what He did for me (and for all who choose Him).

My mom was a great flower gardener. Quite frankly, she could have been a Master Gardener. Each spring, she would get her tools and gloves, put on her summer blouse—in my mind the blouse is always blue—and then plan out her flower garden. So attired and prepared for outside work, Mom would be outside for hours planting her flowers. One spring day, one of those perfect spring days in which the sun was shining and the chill of the night was not quite out of the air early in the morning, I woke up early from a dream.

Most of the dream was incredibly vivid and remains so to this day, over four decades later. The dream began with my mom, dad, and brother watching TV in the living room. In the dream, I walked out of the laundry room into the kitchen, which overlooked the living room. As I walked into the kitchen, I could see my dad sitting in his recliner, facing the TV, which was not an unusual place for Dad to be. What was unusual was the Man standing next to his chair. This Man stood on the opposite side of Dad from me in a place where there should have been no room for Him to stand. Dad's chair was close to a wall with only a side table holding the ashtray between the chair and the wall. This Man was standing where the side table was typically positioned.

In the dream, I stopped and stared at this strange Man who stared back at me. I was not afraid of the Man; I was just surprised. Then He smiled and I smiled, and that is all I remember of the dream. Of the Man, I clearly remember the smile, but the rest of Him is too fuzzy to describe. When I awoke, I immediately wanted to tell someone, so I went looking for Mom. She was outside working on her flower garden.

I went outside in my pjs and told her my dream. She paused for a moment, taking a glove off to massage her left hand. Even back then, her arthritis was starting up. Mom asked, "Who do you think He was?"

I paused a moment and answered, "He was that Man up on the cross." This surprised her, I could tell, so I quickly added, "The one from church."

Mom smiled and said, "What a nice dream." Nothing more was said, but I had shared the dream. Duty done, I went back inside and got a bowl of cereal, Cap'n Crunch, if I remember correctly.

I am not claiming this dream was a visitation as some would believe. It may or may not have been. What I do know is even then, at five years old, I knew who Jesus was and how He had died on a cross similar to the one I saw every Sunday at our Methodist church. To me, early on, Jesus was and is alive.

Chapter 1

When did you first hear about Jesus?

Is He alive to you, even now? Or is He unknown to you?

1 Timothy 4:12 (ESV): "Let no one despise you for your youth, but set the believers an example in speech, in conduct, in love, in faith, in purity."

Chapter 2

I wish I could say in my teens and twenties I had lived my life as a follower of Christ. I did not. I call my time in college "the lost years," and when I was in high school, I am convinced I was three-quarters crazy. Some people reading this may remember me in my high school years. If any of you reading this have been hurt or offended by my self-destructive behavior, I am sorry. I apologize.

Today, I understand that puberty hit, and my testosterone went from zero to a thousand in a few days, so I probably was clinically crazy for a while. Additionally, I was exposed to porn at 12 years old and was struggling through that mess. I was also dealing with an older person whose interest in me was illegal, immoral, and downright evil, meaning I was struggling emotionally, physically, and spiritually. I am not making an excuse, but only describing a reality. I did not have the day-to-day wisdom, control, or discipline I needed to keep in line. None of this is to excuse my behavior. It does not excuse it. I share these facts only to be as transparent as I can be. I still struggle even forty years later with some of the things I had done and some of the stuff done to me, but I can say today I am forgiven. I have forgiven others, and Christ is healing me and making me a new creation. He can do the same for you.

Time. They say time heals all wounds. It did not for me. Time and choices layered calluses on old wounds, which only hid the damage for a great many years. I know some of you reading this understand exactly what I mean. It does not matter what gender, ethnicity, socio-economic group, or religion you may be, personal violation through abuse, whether it be physical, mental, emotional, and/or sexual, is a wound too many carry silently and work hard to cover up and deeply bury. Abuse is a betrayal and is unforgivable, except when Christ comes to free us.

My encouragement to those of you who have had to deal with these things is to pray, to give the offender over to God, to release yourself from the trap of the wound, and to forgive. Forgiveness is a choice. It may be a choice you can make only with God's help, but ultimately you have to choose to forgive and to forgive as often as every day until you can truly set the burden down and not pick it up again.

For those of us who have had to learn to cope, the Apostle Paul teaches in Galatians 6:2a that we should "bear one another's burdens." We need to come alongside each other, pray, commiserate, and encourage each other to fight through this, forgive, and overcome with God's help. Please do not let the offender continue to live in your heart and mind.

If you are reading this and you find yourself in an abusive relationship, get help, and get help now. God does not want this type of relationship for you. Abuse is not in His plan. Seek help and keep seeking help until someone listens and acts.

As a teenager, I did not go to church very often. I went only when it was demanded of me. When I was in college, I almost never went to church, probably less than five times over the course of my college career. I was too busy drinking and sort of studying. Frankly, it is a miracle I graduated from college at all.

I would tell people during these lost years that I was a Christian, but I did not follow Him at all. I did not go to church, and I did not read His Word. I did not pray very much. I did not fellowship or hang out with other believers. What was worse, I did not display any kind of Christian example for my wife. Under my leadership, we spent most of our weekends and many weeknights drinking and carousing together.

Thankfully, I had parents and grandparents who prayed for me and persisted.

Have you ever walked away from God? Are you apart from Him now?

Are you praying for someone who is lost? Are you lost?

Psalms 119:176 (ESV): "I have gone astray like a lost sheep; seek your servant, for I do not forget your commandments."

Chapter 3

I married early. We were twenty-one and had been together for over three years. My wife, Laura, was born a few weeks before me and grew up maybe nine miles from my hometown. Laura's dad owned and ran a TV repair shop back when TVs had tubes and could still be repaired. My parents were regular customers and were friends with my wife's parents back when we were both born. In fact, a week or two after my parents brought me home from the hospital, my future father-in-law was in the house repairing an old TV in the family room. Mom invited him to look in on me as he had been telling my mom about their newest baby, my future wife Laura, who was their seventh child.

I met my wife for the first time when I was around ten years old. Neither of us realized we had met until much later in our lives together. The day we first met, my dad and I went shopping for a new TV. We went shopping in my future father-in-law's shop, and while my dad negotiated TV prices with him, I tried watching a cable channel on one of the TVs in his shop.

I grew up out in the country, and this was well before cable and satellite TV were available in rural areas. In his shop, my future father-in-law had cable TV set up on a single set. At home we had an antenna, which received five channels on a good day.

In his shop, he had a movie channel on, and while they negotiated prices, I watched this crazy movie about a little girl who kept monsters as pets. While watching this weird movie, in the corner of my eye, I caught a shape darting around a corner. I looked up and saw this intense redhead about my own age staring at me with a huge smile on her face. She asked me if I liked the movie. I nodded, and her dad shooed her into the back of the shop to do her homework. Years later, Laura told me that she was definitely that redhead girl.

Laura and I did not meet again until we were seventeen. It's funny. We went to the same schools from seventh grade on. We were in the same grade, and we had our first non-family related or non-farm jobs in the same shopping center. We were close to meeting each other for years, but we never shared a class nor did we meet outside of school until the summer between our junior and senior years.

Then one late summer day, a friend of ours introduced us in the parking lot of my retail job. (Thank you, Jenny!) After we met, we kept running into each other, all over and often—at our college standardized tests, at restaurants, at stores, and at work. Also, for the first time during the fall and spring semesters of our senior year, we had several classes together.

With all of these intersections, we became quick friends and enjoyed being around each other. We were friends for months, and then on prom night right before graduation, we were suddenly more. It took us some time to sort through our friendship turned romance, but I was passionately and madly in love with her, and I have been for over thirty years.

Laura was raised Catholic. I was raised Methodist with some Free Will Baptist thrown in the mix. Neither of us was really sure about our faith. We believed in Jesus, but we did not necessarily trust Him. I know I prayed at times, but my prayers were more like rubbing Buddha's belly. I asked for stuff. I did not understand the difference between believing in Him and fully trusting Him. Laura did not either.

We eventually went to college together and were married at 21 years of age. Children were important to Laura. She made this fact plain to me one night on a date. If I did not want kids, our relationship would not work for her. I did not want kids back then, but I accepted that we would have them together some day. My plan was to put kids off as long as possible.

After the wedding and after we had graduated from college I took my first big job in retail management. The hours were long and the work required us to move from store to store at least once a year for several years. Laura worked in retail management as well but for a different company. After a few moves from store to store around northern Indiana, we both figured out these moves were not benefitting our careers or our pocketbooks. We always seemed to come out behind financially after every move. The cost of moving was always higher than we ever were reimbursed for, and the salary increases were always lower than the cost of living increases in the new areas we moved to; basically we lost money every time we moved. So, we decided to take a risk and choose to move cross country from Indiana to Arizona.

What is the biggest risk you ever took?

Was it a leap of faith or were you completely self-reliant?

How did it work out?

Isaiah **43:18–19** (ESV): "Remember not the former things, nor consider the things of old. Behold, I am doing a new thing; now it springs forth, do you not perceive it? I will make a way in the wilderness and rivers in the desert."

Chapter 4

Throughout our marriage, Laura and I had taken several vacations out West, and we both loved Arizona, especially the town of Flagstaff. When we decided to move, we chose Flagstaff and began discussing with our employers a transfer to the West. It turned out the company I worked for at the time had a pressing need for a retail executive in their northern Arizona store location. Laura's company did as well, so we both had jobs prior to our move to Flagstaff. Even better, and thankfully, my company agreed to pay for our move west. God was blessing us; we had jobs, and our move was paid for, including a flight out to find housing.

At the time of the move, we lived in "the Region," an area in northwestern Indiana right by Chicago. The Region is the local name for the greater northwestern Indiana Chicago suburbs. Our jobs at the time were very difficult and we worked long hours without seeing much of each other.

Our long hours made it especially difficult to get any extra time off. To help get the needed time off to find housing, we both worked twelve-plus hour days for six or seven days in a row. This allowed us to take a long weekend so we could take a flight out to Arizona and find a place to live in Flagstaff. We scheduled our flight in mid-January of 2000 with our eventual move scheduled for February 2000.

Our work schedules prevented us from spending quality time with each other or with our families. Whenever we did have time or found the energy to make the drive, we stayed at my parents' house or at her parents' house. The Region is roughly ninety minutes away from where we both grew up. Whenever we went to my parents, I would spend part of the time target shooting. The precision and the focus I needed to be accurate helped clear my mind of the stress of working retail. I have always been a decent shot with a rifle, and I was bound and determined to get better at shooting with a pistol.

Two weekends before our Arizona flight, we visited my parents as well as Laura's folks. We each packed an overnight bag separately. I always packed a duffel bag we had purchased in Hawaii. It was blue with "HAWAII" in bold white letters on the side. I liked this bag as it was a deep duffle with many side pockets for toiletries.

Besides my clothes and toiletries, I packed a pistol for shooting practice and put it in the side compartment of my Hawaii bag. I liked keeping the pistol in the side compartment as it ensured it would not get mixed into the rest of the junk. Plus, it was secure there. One time, I had packed it in the same side pocket with my toiletries, and it took me a few days to get the toothpaste out of the firearm's action.

At our apartment, I kept the pistol in a secure drawer in our bedroom. After we made this trip to my parents, instead of securing the pistol in the side drawer, I left it in the side compartment of the Hawaii bag. In the days leading up to the flight to Flagstaff, the pistol would come to mind a few times throughout the week. Every time the pistol came to mind, I would remind myself, *When you get home, put the pistol away.* I never did.

Our flight to Flagstaff was early on a Friday morning. We were flying out of Midway Airport. While the mileage from our apartment to Midway was only about 50 miles, it was a 90-minute drive with Chicago traffic. The Thursday before our flight, both Laura and I worked inconvenient shifts. I was a "mid," meaning

I'd get home about 8:00–9:00 p.m. after a twelve-hour day. Laura closed, so she'd be home after midnight.

Both of us had worked all of those twelve-hour days in a row. We were both exhausted and decided to pack in the morning. We set our alarms and crashed. Both of us slept straight through our alarms and woke in a panic. We had no time for showers or detailed packing. So we threw clothes in random bags and tossed in toiletries before racing down to the car. Laura drove as she was the NASCAR driver of the family back then.

We had a little over two hours to get to the airport with no time to check a bag. We would have to take our bags as carry-on luggage. If we hit the airport right, we would have thirty minutes to get from the parking garage to the gate. This was back in early 2000, well before 9/11 and all of the airline security changes. Everything was different back then. Thirty minutes may have been enough time to make it through security and to the gate. We never found out.

Laura drove as fast as the car and traffic allowed. At one point, we bottomed the car out sailing over a set of railroad tracks. I kept an eye out for gas leaks behind us. I thought we had ruptured the fuel tank, but everything held. The car was old but steady. We zoomed our way to Midway Airport, parked, and ran into the airport. The entire trip was a bit of a blur, just a near panic the entire time, worrying about missing our flight.

We ran into the airport and up to the security checkpoint. We put our bags on the conveyor belt and got in line to go through the metal detector. I recall looking at my watch thinking that we had 20 minutes. The plane was still boarding, so we might just make it.

About the end of that thought, one of the security personnel asked, "Whose bag is this?"

I looked over, and it was the blue Hawaii bag. It was mine. I raised my hand and said, "It's mine." As soon as I raised my hand, I realized what they had found. A cold hard knot of fear entered my gut, and I felt a keen sense of inevitability.

The security personnel pulled me over nicely and showed me what was on their screen. Pointing to the object on the screen, they asked if the object was what they thought it was. I assured them it was indeed a small pistol. They asked for permission to open the bag, which I did allow. They opened each zipper before opening the final side pocket that contained the pistol.

Withdrawing it from the bag, security checked and found the pistol had a loaded clip. They showed the pistol to me and asked again, "Is this yours, sir?"

I simply nodded numbly yes.

What is the biggest mistake you've ever made?

Was God trying to get your attention?

What was the result?

Numbers 32:23b (ESV): "Be sure your sin will find you out."

1 John 1:9 (ESV): "If we confess our sins, he is faithful and just and will forgive us our sins and purify us from all unrighteousness."

Chapter 5

Obviously, we never made it to Arizona that day. After a perp walk from security to the holding area inside the airport, we—or I should say I—spent most of the morning being processed at the airport. Laura waited outside the holding area. Once processed, I was transferred to a local holding cell in Cook County.

I remember three things quite clearly. First, the holding area was not an actual cell. It was an office with security bars bolted onto the wall. The security team had to handcuff me to the bar to keep me restrained. Secondly, I distinctly remember the look on Laura's face when she saw me handcuffed to the wall, which is a look I will not forget. And thirdly, I recall how professional, polite, and even nice the security folks were throughout the entire ordeal. The security team could have made it incredibly difficult, but instead they were actually kind. I appreciated their kindness and their professionalism very much.

Once I was transferred to the Cook County detention area, I was put in a cell in the back of a local police station. The cell itself was maybe 10 feet by 10 feet. It had a sink, a toilet, and two slabs hanging off the wall, which were facsimiles of beds. The biggest problem I faced in the holding cell was a lack of toilet paper. After the stress of being arrested, perp walked, and processed, no toilet paper was problematic, to say the least (I carry a handkerchief to this day). The lack of food, soap, or palatable drinking water was secondary to there being no TP. It truly was a simple holding cell where I spent over half a day.

There was a great deal of confusion as to what to do with me. Of the two infractions I was being charged with, one charge had been, up until the previous month, a felony. A local judge had overturned the felony law on a technicality, so no one was quite sure if I would be charged with a felony or a misdemeanor.

The confusion over this meant I ended up staying in the holding cell about 16 hours as the local police worked to figure it out. If I were charged with a felony, I would go to the county lockup where I would stay until the following Monday when an attorney would be assigned and a judge would release me. A misdemeanor meant I could get released that day. Thankfully, after a shift change at the jail cell, my wife was able to talk to the desk sergeant and get me released after midnight.

Of course, I did not understand any of this at the time. I was in shock, I suppose. How could I have been so incredibly stupid and reckless? As the cell door shut in front of me, the gravity of the incarceration and what it might mean for our future was crushing me.

Panic welled up inside me and choked me. It was hard to breathe as terrible thought followed terrible thought. Would I be going to prison? I was in lockup already. Once I went through a trial, would I go to actual prison? I had tried taking a pistol on an airplane for goodness' sake—what kind of jail time would I be looking at? And once released from the holding cell, would I be allowed to leave the state of Illinois? How does the justice system work? What about Arizona? Would we be able to go? Would we be able to move there? What about work? What if they found out?

The weight of worry started out as a fairly large pebble in my shoe, but when it started rolling, it kept rolling and went downhill fast, gathering muck the whole way. The pebble moved fast and turned into this immense crushing boulder of fear. For the first time in a very long time, I turned to prayer. I stood facing the bars of the cell and begged God to get me out of this.

My prayer was incredibly self-centered, entirely all about me and my worry, and focused only on what I wanted. *Get me out of this, Lord! This can't happen to ME! How could it? I don't deserve this!* I do not even remember all of the dross I poured out, which mimicked a poor excuse for a prayer. The prayer did not last very long, though, as conviction poured into me.

By conviction, I mean it in a Christian sense, not the traditional legal system sense of the word. This kind of conviction is when the Holy Spirit instills in us a sense of our own wrongness as compared to how God sees us or wants us to be. It is not as a friend of mine once called an external guilt trip or a "Biblical beatdown," although it can feel that way. Instead, at least for me, conviction is a thought more along the lines of "You are better than this" or "You can be better than this." As Jesus says in John 16:18 (ESV), "And when He [the Holy Spirit] comes, He will convict the world concerning sin and righteousness and judgment." In the previous verse, Jesus describes the Holy Spirit as a "Helper." This conviction was the Holy Spirit trying to help me.

God, through the Holy Spirit, was telling me that He wanted more from me than selfish foxhole-type prayers. I stopped my faux prayer and just listened. Do not get me wrong—I was not hearing voices in my head; I was feeling convicted and sensing the wrongness in me. I was listening to this feeling of wrongness. I walked away from the bars and sat on the edge of the pseudo "bed." I put my head in my hands, and after a while, I started to pray a true prayer.

This time my prayer was right. I was positionally correct. I was the one in error. I was in the wrong and had been for quite a long time. I had accepted Christ as my Savior years ago, but I had not behaved as if I really trusted Him with my life. Oh, I trusted that when I died I would spend eternity with Him, and rightly so. I simply was not living as if I trusted Him with this life, the here and now. I was not living as if I loved Him. Sitting in the jail cell, and recalling how I had reacted to being jailed, made it abundantly clear to me that I was not right with the Lord.

So, I prayed. I confessed my sins to Him. I asked that His will be done with this arrest, and I asked Him to give me the strength to deal with whatever was to come. I put my full faith and trust in Him for the first time. I probably prayed like this for over 30 minutes. When I was through, I was at peace. As the Apostle Paul wrote in Philippians 4:7 (ESV): "And the peace of God, which surpasses all understanding, will guard your hearts and minds in Christ Jesus."

After this prayer, I slept for most of the sixteen hours I was in the cell. Laura was able to talk to the night shift supervisor who took a look at my arrest and what I was to be charged with, and he released me shortly after midnight. We spent the rest of the night in a local hotel and then drove home to Indiana the next morning. There were plenty of messages waiting for me from our family.

I learned later that my mom had to rush my dad to the ER to get him medication to calm his nerves. He had been calling the jail, apparently every hour, and was a bit of a wreck. When we talked, he was fine and I assured him that all was well with me. He had found a couple of attorneys for me so we called one on Monday and made an appointment to go see him.

Laura and I both liked and trusted the attorney and paid his retainer. I was to be charged with two misdemeanors, and after receiving the retainer, he put his researchers to work on the case. We were free to move to Arizona. We just needed to make sure we appeared in court in 30 days; otherwise, I would never be able to set foot in the city of Chicago again.

Eventually, Laura and I made the move to Arizona. Online, Laura found an apartment complex close to the stores we were going to work in. We rented the two-bedroom/two-bath apartment without seeing it. We worked with a moving company, got everything packed, and then drove ourselves across the country. It was a fun trip even though the arrest was hanging over me.

When we arrived in Flagstaff, we got right to work. Retail is not the type of job that allows for extended time off, even during slow sales periods. We quickly assimilated into the store cultures and into the culture of the northern Arizona community. We love the area to this day and often vacation there.

I started reading my Bible regularly as well as works by Christian authors. A favorite author of mine is C.S, Lewis, with two of his influential books *Mere Christianity* and *God in the Dock* being essential for me. Indeed, C.S. Lewis has left an indelible mark on me. Through his writings he made it clear to me that Christianity is not just a religion, or just a faith, or only a relationship; it is also an education. If we believe in Him, trust in Him, and want to be more like Him, we have to learn about Him, and the only way to do that is through His Word, and through teaching, preaching, and sharing His Word.

After my arrest, and my trusting in Him for the first time, I began to consume Christian writings and scripture like food at a smorgasbord. I had no real structure or system to my consumption; I grabbed whatever I could, wherever I could, whenever I could and read it.

Laura and I still were not going to church. She was raised Catholic and I was raised Methodist, for the most part, so we had never found a church that fit both of our expectations. This was a poor excuse; church was just something that would take time for us to come around on.

During our settling-in period, we flew back to Chicago twice to finish up the legal issues. Our attorney, God bless him, had found a technical issue in my arrest. His plan was to use this technicality to have the charges dropped. He believed my packing of the gun was completely unintentional, and he found an issue in the charges that he believed he could use for my benefit. He was doing everything he could to defend me. At first, I thought, *Yes! let's find a way to get these charges dropped or thrown out.* At first.

Then, I thought more about it in the light of my faith. I did actually commit the crime. I did not mean to commit it, but ignorance is no excuse. I was not sure what to do, so I prayed. A simple answer kept coming back, no matter how I prayed. The answer was to avoid loopholes—no trickery, no shortcuts, no technicalities. I did it; I had to stop trying to force things and trust God. I called my attorney back in Chicago, talked it through with him, and told him I would let him know at our next court appearance.

Laura and I discussed what I was thinking, and she agreed with me. As much as neither of us wanted me to have a criminal record, we also did not want to betray our faith. We decided the best action would be to have our lawyer get us the best deal possible without any legal jujitsu.

We flew back to Chicago for our last court date. We met our attorney outside the courtroom and told him what we wanted. He was definitely perplexed but agreed to do what we asked. He approached the prosecutor and they met with the judge. Together they came up with an agreement. I would stand in court, the charges would be read aloud, the judge would issue a judgment of one year of probation, and I would be free to go.

I cannot describe the relief I felt walking out of the courtroom after three months of working through our legal system. I had been arrested in Chicago at Midway airport in January of 2000, and we finished up the court proceedings by the end of March that year. All in all, we probably spent over four thousand dollars in fees, expenses, and fines. I have two misdemeanors on my record, although they no longer show up in most background checks as they are now over twenty years old.

It was not a pleasant experience, but it was a necessary one. Sometimes God has to use a 2x4 board to the head to get our attention. If God is trying to get your attention, He will do whatever it takes to get it. He had been after me for years, and I had kept putting Him off. Whenever I hear the parable Jesus tells us about the lost sheep, I think about me. In the parable, the Shepherd of the lost sheep searches until He finds it. The point is the Good Shepherd will not let the stray stay lost.

My friend, if God is trying to get your attention, listen to Him. He is not going to give up. He won't run out of time, although we humans do run out of time. He will come for His lost sheep. He will pursue you until you make a decision. Don't wait. He is trying to help you!

I have one more reason on why we chose to seek a plea deal rather than pursue the technicality approach. During one of my prayers about the decision, I saw a crystal clear image in my mind of the future me talking to my son (even though I didn't have a son at the time). We were discussing responsibility and accountability, and I could not shake the thought that if I took the easy way, the worldly way, the "technicality" way out of the mess I was in, I would not have a leg to stand on in talking about responsibility or accountability with any future children.

Have you ever felt convicted?

How did you respond?

Is Jesus reaching out to you now?

Luke 15:4 (ESV): "Suppose one of you has a hundred sheep and loses one of them. Doesn't he leave the ninety-nine in the open country and go after the lost sheep until he finds it?"

Chapter 6

Once the legal mess was put to bed, Laura and I settled into life in Flagstaff. Flag is a mountain town placed at the crossroads to the Grand Canyon. It sits about seven thousand feet above sea level. It is one of the few places in Arizona that experiences all four seasons, and all four of those seasons have plenty of sunshine. The average sunshine is three hundred days of the year.

Flag is a tourist town as well as a college town; it is home to Northern Arizona University. Most of the people who live there come from somewhere else. And as a retirement community, at least when we lived there, Flag also had an unusually high number of master's degrees strewn amongst its population. The town has a high population of well-educated people. After we settled into the community and started to get to know a diverse group of friends, Laura and I quickly realized we could be having dinner at a local eatery and the owner and server could be a former VP who was restructured out of his job and started a business just for the fun of it.

The hiking, the views, and the outdoor culture of the town were such that even though our jobs demanded a lot of hours, we spent as much free time as we could hiking up and down Mt. Humphrey's or Mt. Elden, or for a light workout we would hike Buffalo Park. We were getting into the best shape of our lives, which ended up being a great thing for both of us.

About a year after moving to Flagstaff, Laura put a deadline on having our first baby. By this time, we had been married eight years and were quickly approaching age thirty. The biological clock was ticking, so we finally agreed to start trying in December of 2000. I was ambivalent at best, but I knew a baby was what she wanted, so I put my trust in Christ for His timing, thinking He may not want us to have kids for a long while.

As is often the case for me, God's plans and timing are much bigger and on a different timeline than I usually want or even imagine. I suppose the only thing limiting God is my lack of faith. Whenever I just relax and truly trust Him, life is always much better, much more fun (eventually), and far more adventurous.

We started trying in December and we were pregnant just after New Year's. God had to be laughing at me. I have no doubt He was rewarding Laura's faithfulness. Notice I said "we" were pregnant. When Laura got pregnant, I was as involved as I could be. I could not carry the baby, but I could carry my wife when she needed me. It was during this pregnancy that she started calling me her "water nazi." No matter where she was or what she was doing, I would call her cell and make sure she was drinking plenty of water. I was also on her about a healthy diet, vitamins, and exercise, besides her water intake. We wanted her and this pregnancy, our baby, to have every chance of being as successful and healthy as possible. At the altitude in which we lived, dehydration can be quick, so hydration was all important to keep them both healthy.

Around the four-month mark of the pregnancy, we had a definite scare. Laura and I had gone off-roading in our 4x4 truck down in the Red Rock country of Sedona. The area we drove in had flooded a few weeks prior. Other people with four-wheel drive trucks had gone through mudding, leaving deep tire tracks all over the back road. When the mud dried under the Arizona sun, what was left were a series of deep rough tire ruts. Driving down the back road, we bounced around like steel balls in an old pinball machine throughout the drive. We had taken drives like this one all the previous year, so we did not think a whole lot about it.

The next day at work, Laura called me, obviously distressed. She was spotting or showing some blood, which is not a very good sign when one is pregnant. Laura called while she was driving to our ob-gyn. I quickly told my boss I had to leave. I jumped into my truck and made the three-mile drive in about five minutes, which isn't bad, considering I had to drive through downtown to get to the doctor.

Laura was in a back room of the doctor's office waiting for the doctor when I arrived. I was ushered back and everyone was quite serious. This was our first baby, and you never know how these things will turn out. It was at this point I realized I was going to be a father, and it meant far more to me than I ever realized. The baby who was in Laura's womb was as real to me as any human being I knew who was up and walking around. And I didn't want to lose him.

Laura and I held each other as we waited for our ob-gyn. We did not say anything. We just sat and held each other. The doctor came in and got to work. Thankfully, everything was fine. We had put too much stress on Laura driving over and bouncing up and down those bloody ruts. The doctor gave me the most withering of looks when we confessed what we had done that weekend. I can still feel the heat of it today. (And I deserved the look.)

The rest of the pregnancy went extremely well. Our son was born in late September, a little early and weighing less than seven pounds, which is typical for babies born at high altitude. His thin frame filled out very quickly, and within a few months he became an infant version of the Michelin man, rolls upon rolls of fat that bounced with every step.

Bringing him home the first time was absolutely terrifying for both of us. I am quite certain we annoyed the heck out of the nurses at the medical facility. If our son coughed or made a weird noise, the call button was hit. If Laura was in the shower and he needed a diaper change, the call button was hit. If he gurgled oddly or would not breastfeed, the button was hit. I am quite certain the nursing staff was happy to send us on our way.

The first night with our son at home, I experienced overwhelming love, pride, a new sense of purpose, as well as, quite frankly, abject fear. But I also knew God was giving us a heritage and it was up to us, up to me I felt, as to what our heritage would be. Would we have a heritage of the world or of God?

How do you view children, as a blessing or something else?

Do you view adoption as a viable option? Why or why not?

What legacy are you leaving?

Psalm 127:3 (ESV): "Behold, children are a heritage from the Lord, the fruit of the womb a reward."

Chapter 7

After our son was born, many, many family members came to visit us. We appreciated all of the visits, all of them, even if it meant our small apartment was packed full for a while. I had several weeks of vacation saved up at work. I took as many weeks off as policy allowed (three weeks) so I was able to spend time and bond with our son every single day for those precious three weeks. The Sunday before I was set to go back to work, I felt a compelling desire to go back to church.

I had been avoiding church. I had no good reason really, just a small incident from when I was younger that I used it as an excuse. During my teen years I went, for a short while, to a fiery well-intentioned church. The church had a lot of energy, a lot of people my age, and it focused on the works side of our faith.

By works, I mean they liked demonstrations, usually emotional, of everyone's commitment to Christ. If there were no tears every other Sunday, people thought something was wrong. Now, tears are fine when they are genuine. But an expectation of tears every other worship service tends to lead people, at least it did for me, to a false show. Every Sunday, at the end of the service and after the message had been delivered, there was an altar call. An altar call is when the pastor invites worshipers to come up to the front, kneel at the altar, and pray in response to the sermon.

This is how I interpreted the altar call: if I were serious about my Christianity, any time there was an altar call, I'd better go up. So,

I went up every Sunday for three Sundays in a row. Then on the fourth Sunday, it occurred to me I was going up to the altar to be seen, not because I felt God leading me or I was feeling convicted by the sermon. I was going up entirely for show. I was being fake in my religiosity.

Jesus made a hard point about this idea of being seen by others. In Matthew 23:5a, He said, "They do all their deeds to be seen by others." This section of scripture, chapter 23, is known as the Seven Woes. Jesus was lambasting the religious leaders of His day. "For they preach, but do not practice." He was assailing them for being false. I was no different when I went up to the altar so I could be seen. I was being false.

After that particular Sunday, I left the church and did not go back, other than for an occasional visit every few years. I am still friends with people who were in that church with me. My putting on a show was my own fault, no one else's, and certainly not theirs. Now, twenty years after this event, the physical presence of my son, and the knowledge that his education and his knowledge of Christ sat squarely on my shoulders, were motivating me. Laura and I agreed that while we would always make decisions together, ultimately our faith or lack thereof was my responsibility.

About this time, my grandfather and I had a talk about church and how important it was, and his recommendation was to go somewhere that would not be too fiery but not too Catholic, either. So we went through the phone book and found a church that was a conglomeration of three distinct denominations with members from Protestant and Catholic backgrounds.

We decided to attend this church on a day that happened to be World Music Sunday. What an amazing worship service. At the time—maybe it still is—the choir was conducted by and staffed with faculty and students from Northern Arizona University. NAU is a great school all around, and they have an exceptional music program. We were treated to a Sunday service filled with gospel music from around the globe. It was a beautiful and stirring worship service.

The sermon that day was on Ezekiel 22:30, "And I sought for a man among them who should build up the wall and stand in the breach before me for the land, that I should not destroy it, but I found none." With our new son, I was terrified I would lead him away from God, and here I was hearing a message about how followers of Christ need to stand in the gap for God. I did not really understand what was meant by standing in the breach or gap for God, but it greatly affected me. The message and the worship service spoke to both of us. We had found our church. The church became a family for us, and I met one of the most important spiritual leaders in my life, Pastor Bill Van Loan.

Was church a part of your childhood or is it new to you?

What do you expect from your church family?

What does God want you to do as it relates to church?

Hebrews 13:7 (ESV): "Remember your leaders, those who spoke to you the word of God. Consider the outcome of their way of life, and imitate their faith."

Chapter 8

We became regular attenders of our church. The worship music continued to be an excellent part of each service. The church was in the midst of a pastoral change, and one of the denominations had sent an interim pastor to help them transition away from a long-term pastor and prepare for a new permanent pastor.

The interim pastor position is a very special role and takes a very special kind of minister of God. Interim pastors usually step into a situation where a pastor has left on bad terms or after a very long time in the position, sometimes as long as twenty-plus years. These interim pastors know they are temporary (maybe a year or two at most) and have to deal with feelings of sadness, anger, disappointment, or even relief. They help the congregation take stock of where they are as a congregation and to discern where God is leading them. They do all of this with intensity and fervor, knowing they will need to leave in a short while. And when they leave, they really leave, cutting ties with leadership to smooth the way for the incoming leader.

Pastor Bill was an interim pastor. His sermons were biblical, pointed, and always grounded in the Gospel. In the church, broadly speaking, there is a term known as "stepping on toes." It is used when the pastor preaches a sermon that seems to be aimed right at you personally, and it hits you where you live. It feels as if the pastor is about to call you out by name and tell everyone your secret (or not so secret) sin. It hurts, it is uncomfortable, and no one really likes it when it happens, especially me. Interim pastors "step on toes" to help the congregation grow.

For a very long time, probably as long as I can remember, I struggled with pride and lust. I've gotten a heckuva lot better on the lust front, but I have to be very careful. I do not even look at the covers of magazines at the checkout line in stores anymore. Pride, on the other hand, is one I struggle with in an on-again, off-again relationship. Unfortunately, pride can be more on-again than I care to admit.

I was still early in my spiritual formation, and I was hiking and reading the Bible a lot. I did not really understand scripture most of the time. Pastor Bill's weekly sermons were helpful as they were grounded in the Word and helped me to understand what God was trying to tell us in certain passages. It was the rest of the time that I struggled.

At work, I was able to get a set day off, which in retail is a relief. I had every Thursday off for years. Scheduling appointments and long hikes all became a lot easier once I was able to get a set day off. Laura had not gone back to her retail job. Instead, through our Flagstaff community network, Laura was able to connect with a local artist and began working out of her home. (Thank you, Judy!) The artist was gracious enough to allow Laura to take our son to work with her. Her job and the artist were a massive blessing to us.

On a particular Thursday, I was watching our son and decided to go for a walk downtown. I was pushing our son along in a stroller and happened to run into Pastor Bill. He was walking downtown to go to lunch. (Flag has outstanding local eateries; a food tour of Flagstaff is worth the effort.) He invited me to go with him, so the three of us sat down and started to get to know each other.

We spent the next few weeks and months becoming friends. Pastor Bill helped me to understand the basic tenets of the faith, gave me the tools to read and understand scripture, and helped guide my growth in the faith. He helped answer some hard questions I was struggling with, including some technical questions. For example, my maternal grandmother, Helen, was struggling with Alzheimer's. This disease affected the entire family. I knew Grandma was a woman of faith so I was not concerned for her eternal destination, but I wondered what happens to people who are in those situations in which their mind is deteriorating.

I asked him during one of our walks, and he took a long time to answer. I discovered later on that this was a question he had struggled with in his own personal life. His answer went something like this: As a mind deteriorates, the world falls away, and people who are in this sort of state of mind, their mind is going and the world is going away with it. In those circumstances, Christ can become more apparent to them—more real than ever before. The less they are of the world, the closer they can be to Him. This hinges, of course, on whether they knew Christ before they became ill. I found a great deal of comfort in his answer.

Over the spring and summer of 2002, Pastor Bill and I had several deep conversations. We had him over for dinner, and we had lunch together numerous times. He introduced me to several church members who were instrumental in helping me grow spiritually as well. Regardless of topic, circumstance, or questions, the pastor or church members kept pointing me back to either Christ or to scripture. And for followers to grow, I believe this technique is fundamental. Regardless of which church tradition you come from, or maybe you don't come from a church tradition at all, a fundamental truth is the Bible, scripture, is God's Word to us. He is literally talking to us through His Word. And when we need to hear from Him, His Word stands ready.

I believe scripture is God's spoken word written down and put there for us to hear Him speak directly to us. I do not mean I interpret scripture for my own personal use—that should never be done. I do not mean that at all. What I mean is when we want or need God to speak to us, we must turn to scripture. What should we do in a particular circumstance? What should we believe?

Where should we go? In His Word, if we read it, study it, and believe it, He has answers for us.

We may not like those answers because sometimes the answer is No, or Not Yet, or Wait. We, especially me, like instant gratification. I love on-demand movies or TV shows! God, however, does not always provide on-demand answers. Sometimes we have to wait, even a lifetime, to understand what He is doing. Sometimes He does provide the instant answer. And I will caution when He does start to move, He can come like a hurricane, all at once and seemingly from every direction. He is God, after all.

Besides working with Laura and me on becoming members of the church and baptizing me, Pastor Bill also baptized our son. I had the privilege of being baptized with my son on the same day. It is a tradition in the church that when a father is baptized, the whole household can be baptized with him, so that is what we did. It was beautiful and touching. As a Catholic, Laura was baptized at birth and committed herself to Christ during the same service.

Right after becoming members, we joined a Sunday school class at the church, which became, and still is, an extended part of our family to this day, nearly twenty years later. Our class became our life group. Life groups are a group of people who become your mutual friends, your mutual advisors, your mutual support, people who go through life with you, hand in hand. They become your core network with everyone helping each other out as needed.

This Sunday school group became our core support team, which we would need soon enough. In addition, an older expat couple adopted us as their extended family, and we spent all of our holidays with them. Some couples were about our age. We golfed together, lunched together, hung out together, supported each other, and loved each other. This group and a group at another church in Flagstaff helped carry us through what was to come.

How are you growing spiritually?

What practices are you engaging in? Prayer, reading, meditation....?

How can your church family help you to grow?

Proverbs 11:14 (ESV): "Where there is no guidance, a people falls, but in an abundance of counselors there is safety."

Chapter 9

My son celebrated his first birthday in September of 2002. We had
a big party and thoroughly enjoyed ourselves. It was, quite literally,
the calm before the storm. The weekend after his first birthday,
Laura was working at an official AKC dog show. Laura, through
her work with the local artist, had become involved in a nonprofit,
focused on the very active and very passionate dog community in
Flagstaff. Because of this work, she participated in local AKC events
to raise funds.

Our son stayed home with me while she worked the show. I was
off on this particular Saturday. Early that morning, I woke up
and felt tired and physically off. My lower back had been sore
for days. Feeling exhausted the day after a long shift at the end
of a long week was not unusual. About mid-morning, I began to
develop a migraine and took a couple generic pills. Whenever I get
a migraine, other than sleep, pain relievers—which are a mixture
of aspirin, acetaminophen, and caffeine—were the only drugs that
could affect the migraine. I took two, trying to forestall the attack. I
waited an hour and took another one.

The morning dragged on as I physically deteriorated. At noon, I
was set to feed my son lunch. I heated up his all-natural macaroni
and cheese, opened peaches, and set up some breast milk for him.
Unusually for him, he did not want to eat. Nothing I put in front
of him would satisfy him. He was in a mood and did not want
anything. He kept "squawking," half crying, half grunting. I was not

feeling well and was feeling sicker with each passing second. My stomach was churning, my head hurt, and I was cranky myself. I recall having a heated argument with my one-year-old, which made him cry big hitching, sobbing tears.

After the one-sided argument, I felt awful physically as well as emotionally because I had made him cry. The churning in my stomach transitioned to a pain in my abdomen, a sharp and nearly unbearable pain. While my son was still in his high chair, I called Laura. I was not going to make it. I was not going to be able to watch him. I figured I had the flu or something. She answered her cell and could tell something was wrong immediately. She came home fairly quickly and I went to bed.

Over the next two days, I struggled with a level of pain that was staggering in its intensity. When I am working, or have a responsibility I am committed to, I can continue to fight an illness, push on through, and fulfill my obligation. This was different, far different from any illness I had felt in the past.

Once I went to bed, I stopped fighting. I stopped fighting whatever was going on inside me, and pain settled in for a long stay. With the pain came a feeling of wrongness. This feeling of wrongness is difficult to explain. The only way I know how to convey this feeling is to compare it to a much smaller previous injury.

When I was sixteen years old, I dislocated my left shoulder. It was really just a stupid accident. While my shoulder was dislocated, my arm would work, but not very well. I could lift my arm only so high and turn it only slightly. My arm was out of joint, and the dislocation felt entirely wrong. The pain of the dislocation was high but focused only in the joint. Even at sixteen, the pain was not as bad as the feeling of wrongness, being out of joint. The pain was secondary to righting the wrong of the dislocation. So I popped the shoulder back in myself, teeth gritted through the pain.

Back in 2002, on this night, my entire body felt completely out of joint, and there was nothing I could do to correct it myself. I just had to lie there and take it, the wrongness and the pain. When Laura came to bed that night, exhausted herself from a long day, I moved into the TV room. I lay on the living room floor praying. The pain was constant and consistently high. Every so often my abdomen would spasm, which felt like a total body cramp or charley horse.

My body hurt from my toenails to the hairs on my head. I ran my hand through my sweat-soaked hair, and the movement felt as if I were pulling individual hairs out by the roots. The center of the pain was in my abdomen and back. My diaphragm and my back muscles spasmed over and over and over. Even when they released, they were still tense and quickly tightened again. It felt as if the muscles were tearing themselves apart.

This kept up all night and into most of the next day until my body basically stopped functioning. I did not eat, drink, go to the bathroom, nothing really. Laura and our son were out most of that Sunday. When she got home, Laura finally asked about going to the hospital. I told her no. Stupidly, I said no. The main learning point for me: if I think I should go to the hospital, I should go. On this Sunday, I thought I should go to the ER, but I did not.

Throughout the previous night and day, I learned to manage pain. My body hurt, and it hurt all over. The spasms had stopped, but the pain persisted. I learned how to manage the pain by accepting it. It was that simple for me. The pain was there, I accepted pain was going to be there, and I set my mind to studying the pain. In so doing, I thought I could control it. The really dumb thing is that by controlling it, I was making things worse for myself. The pain was telling me there was something fundamentally wrong. Instead of doing something about it right away and finding professional help, I waited thirty-six hours.

I was afraid and hoped the pain would pass.

Have you ignored pain? What was the outcome?

What are you afraid of? What are your fears?

Are you a control nut? How successful are you at controlling your life?

Matthew 14:31 (ESV): "Jesus immediately reached out his hand and took hold of him, saying to him, 'O you of little faith, why did you doubt?'"

Chapter 10

While I was writhing in unnecessary pain, I prayed over and over for healing. And when healing did not happen, I prayed for relief from the pain, which was a big fat No, or a Not Yet. So I prayed afresh, and I asked God to show me the source of the pain. Almost immediately, I felt a sensation in one of my testicles that felt as if someone had shoved a dull blade into it. I reached down and held it, making sure I had not somehow managed to stab myself with a needle or something.

While I held it, I thought for the first time of testicular cancer. When the stabbing sensation abated, I steeled myself and felt around down there for any lumps. I could not find any, and I breathed a sigh of relief. Then the pain flared up again, and I stopped thinking about cancer or anything else.

Monday morning came, finally, and I agreed to go to my personal physician. Laura called my general practitioner, who agreed to see me before lunch that very day. At the appointment, my doctor helped me up onto an examination table and began to check me thoroughly. He checked my heart, my lungs, my testicles, my prostate, the whole works. All of it felt fine as could be until he pressed on my abdomen. The pressure on my diaphragm started a fresh round of spasms.

After the thorough examination, my doctor could not find any lumps anywhere. My body was sore all over, so when he poked, prodded, and squeezed, it hurt, but nothing stood out. The pain was high enough that he was convinced something severe was wrong inside, so he recommended a scan.

Laura and I were sent over to the medical imaging center for my scan with the full expectation that I would likely be admitted to the hospital. The scan was an emergency abdominal CT scan. I think after twenty years, the process may have changed. Back in 2002, I was in for an unpleasant surprise. My doctor had warned me the scan might be invasive. Invasive was not the word I would have chosen; a personal violation was more accurate.

After being admitted to our hospital room, Laura and I filled out the extensive paperwork and then waited an hour or two. The nurse in charge of my room kept trying to get a pain med for me prior to the scan. This was my first real clue I should be a tad worried about what was to come. While she was trying to secure a pain med, a medical technician showed up and took me to the CT room. Her accent was thick, as she was visiting from Ethiopia. She was incredibly nice and professional, and I suppose she was very helpful considering what she had to do every day.

After checking to make sure I was who I claimed to be, I was rolled through a set of doors and parked next to several machines in the scanning room. I had already changed into a gown, with nothing on underneath. I was then instructed to lie on my side. My thoughts ran along the lines of what the heck for? The pain was not in my side.

My technician explained what she was about to do as I lay there. She showed me a foot-long object with a bulb at the end. She said it was a balloon, and then she showed me a bag of fluid attached to the wand. After explaining the fluid was a contrast dye so my internal GI tract would be clear on the scan, she explained how the dye was going to be injected into me, and then she did it. This sweet person stepped around behind me and rather roughly inserted the wand up into my rectum. After securing it, she then inflated the balloon bulb so it would not fall out. After ensuring the instrument was firmly ensconced, she pumped a gallon or two of contrast dye up my GI tract. Once full of the dye, they scanned me.

As bad as the insertion was, and as embarrassing as it was to hold onto the wand as a secondary precaution to make sure it did not fall out, the worst part of the procedure was after the scan was completed. Once the radiologist had good pictures, the technician came around again and told me to hold onto the fluid after she removed the wand. After deflating the balloon and yanking out the wand, I had to clench hard and then hop down off a table. Then I had to waddle down a hallway, hoping the closest bathroom was empty, all while not "making a mess." A video of me fast waddling down the hall would be hysterical to see.

After finishing up in the bathroom, which took a very long time, and with the test results being approved, I was rolled back to my room. The room nurse was waiting for me. She apologized for not getting back in time. She fussed all over me and made sure I was "all done getting that stuff out." Once she was sure, she injected me with my first dose of morphine.

I admit, from the first shot of it, I am addicted to morphine. Even now, almost twenty years later, my mouth waters at the thought of it. I spent the next week hooked up to a morphine drip and loved every second of it. I pray I never get it again, or that it becomes easy to obtain. I recently had a diverticulitis attack. Even though it was very painful, I refused morphine. I crave it and enjoy it too much.

With the first shot, my pain did not go away, but I stopped caring about the pain. Maybe this is why I refused morphine later on, as pain is a powerful teacher. Paul reminds believers in 2 Corinthians 1:5: "For as we share abundantly in Christ's sufferings, so through Christ we share abundantly in comfort too." In other words, my suffering is valuable and allows me to comfort others who are suffering.

I hold onto Paul's words and the following verse as a promise, conditional on our relationship with Him, that He will one day wipe out all pain.

What promise of God do you hold onto?

How do you keep track of promises God has proven to you?

How do you deal with pain? What are your pain management techniques?

Revelation 21:4 (ESV): "He will wipe away every tear from their eyes, and death shall be no more, neither shall there be mourning, nor crying, nor pain anymore, for the former things have passed away."

Chapter 11

While I floated on the hospital bed in a morphine-induced euphoria, a series of nurses and doctors came in and out. They were always checking vitals, not having much information to share, and were sharing an encouraging word every now and then. Eventually the man who would be my surgeon came in to review with me what they had found on the scan and the plan to deal with the results.

I was expecting—maybe hoping is a better word—that the results would show I had an inflamed or even slightly burst appendix. No matter what it was, everyone was taking it very seriously. The surgeon arrived and talked through what they had found.

The scan/procedure discovered a mass located behind my pancreas roughly the size of a golf ball. The doctors did not know what the mass was, so they had to go in and find out. For me, it meant I was going to have an open exploratory abdominal surgery or a laparotomy. The surgeon was going to open up my abdomen, examine my organs one by one, and then decide what to do with the golf ball-sized mass. The surgery was going to be lengthy and about as invasive as a surgery could get.

The surgery was a major one, and it took a while to get it scheduled. I was put on NPO status. NPO stands for "nil per os," which is Latin. In English, it means "nothing by mouth." I was not allowed to eat or drink until after the surgery. I ended up going three to four days without any food or liquids. I was allowed some neat lemon-flavored cotton swabs to swab out my dry cottonmouth. I loved those lemon swabs.

The surgery was very early on Wednesday. I remember virtually nothing of that morning or the night before, other than praying and lots of morphine. I have a vague recollection of being woken up, and my throat feeling like the Sahara Desert, parched, cracked, and arid. I was then given a shot, and I was aware of nothing more until I woke up well past noon, closer to late afternoon.

With my first surgery, and every surgery afterward, the first thing I always focused on was a clock. My surgery lasted nearly eight hours. When I awoke, my surgeon's nurse practitioner (NP) was standing over me. I will call her Jane. My NP was very nice—sweet, even—but was also very firm—drill sergeant firm. Jane introduced herself and then explained what was going to happen by early evening. She told me, ordered really, that I was going to get out of bed and walk.

I honestly did not believe it would be possible, as my body felt as if it weighed a ton. I also had massive cotton padding covering my abdomen and chest. The cotton pad was disconcerting in its size and thickness. An immense pad of white cotton was taped to my body. Beneath the pad, I imagined I had a "Y" shaped autopsy incision or something similarly large. After checking my vitals, Jane left to check on other patients, but she told me when she came back that she was going to remove the padding.

Laura and our one-year-old son were then allowed to come in to visit me. I was tired and slept through most of their visit. When I was awake again, the NP was back. Jane had help with her and a cart filled with all manner of instruments and bandages.

After setting everything up next to my hospital bed, Jane looked at me intently, ensuring I was focusing on her, and then explained what the surgeon had done and what she was about to do. The surgeon had cut into my abdominal wall from my right side following my rib cage just past my midline, an incision roughly nine inches in length.

When he was finished examining me internally and removing the mass, the surgeon had used over thirty medical staples to seal the incision site and hold it together. The padding was in place to help with any seepage through the staples. I also had a fist-sized plastic bulb attached to two or three feet of medical tubing that was hanging out of my belly. Inside my belly, I had another couple of feet of tubing snaked around inside just beneath the skin. The tubing and the bulb was there to allow for drainage.

Jane warned me when she started to pull the cotton padding back that some of the padding may catch on the staples or on the tubing and it may pull a bit. I should not feel much pain with the morphine, but it could hurt. She was going to go very slowly to make sure she minimized any excess pulling and minimize my pain. Before she started, she asked me if I had any questions.

Jane had been very serious as she explained the process to me. I croaked out, "Just one question." I was still dry and had not been given anything to drink yet.

She sensed something in my tone so she scowled a bit and asked, "Yes?"

"When you pull that back, is anything going to fall out?" I said in a deadpan tone.

Jane burst out laughing with a full throated laugh. She was shocked, to say the least. It was a pleasure to hear the laugh, and the nurse who was with her laughed as well. Humor is my weapon against pain and against difficult times. I laughed a bit as well, but that hurt too much, so I did not laugh long. After our little laugh together, my interactions with Jane were far less formal, and I can say I am very thankful she worked with me on my recovery.

The padding was pulled back slowly for a big dramatic reveal. I was able to see all of those staples for the first time. The skin and staples together looked like a red set of railroad tracks across my abdomen. The visual was surreal. I was still on morphine, so the pain was vague and barely there. This was to change and change quickly, but for the moment, I just took in the sight of it all. Jane gave me a few moments and then began cleaning the area of any post-surgery fluid. She was very gentle and very quick.

Once my chest and abdomen were clean, she gave me her stern look again and said I would be on my feet within 30 minutes. Sure enough, she was right. The floor nurses helped me get out of bed. The incision had cut through my abdominal muscles, so it was almost impossible for me to sit up on my own at the time. They got me up, I walked around a little bit, and then I went back to bed and hit the button on my morphine drip. I slept for hours after my first walk.

My only complaint of the surgery had nothing to do with me. My wife and my son had waited for news during my surgery. They were in a waiting area and spent hours awaiting news. No one from the surgery team came and talked to them after my surgery. It is possible the surgeon had tried to find them and could not; we do not know. She was not paged, either. If you are a medical professional, please make every effort to find the loved ones of your patient.

After the long hours of surgery, Laura started worrying even more than she had been and went looking for answers. She was told I was out of surgery and was back in my room. When she came to see me, it was in relief and anger. We made sure on all future surgeries that the doctor knew where she would be and that they had to find her post-surgery. We made a point of it.

What was your first surgery like?

What concerned you or concerns you about your surgery?

How are you preparing for medical emergencies?

Psalm 41:3 (ESV): "The Lord sustains him on his sickbed; in his illness you restore him to full health."

Chapter 12

After the abdominal surgery, I spent several more days in the hospital recovering. I eventually went off the morphine drip and onto some heavy pain pills. The pain meds helped considerably and were badly needed. The surgeon had opened up my gut, taken all of my organs out, removed the mass, and then put everything back in. I hurt all over. I am thankful for the pain meds and the morphine, but to this day, I minimize and limit how much and how long I take those types of medications. I am more afraid of the pain meds and addiction than of feeling the pain.

Eventually, the surgeon came and visited me to share his findings. After opening me up, he did find the mass. It was the size of a golf ball. Unfortunately, the mass was lying against my inferior vena cava. The vena cava is a large vein that returns blood to the heart from the lower half of the body. The surgeon had removed as much of the mass as he could. He had to leave some of the necrotic tissue inside me, as part of the mass was laying directly on the vena cava. Removing the last bit was extremely dangerous. The surgery had taken longer than expected, and I had lost more blood then was good for me, so instead of risking a major issue by nicking my vena cava, they elected to not scrape the remaining tissue off.

The surgeon was uncertain as to what the mass was, or more accurately, what it had been. The mass, to his trained eye, was mainly black necrotic tissue, or as he explained, dead tissue. Other than dead tissue, he could not tell what the mass had been, as it was nearly gangrenous. The theory is that my body had destroyed whatever the mass had been, and it was rejecting the dead tissue. The rejection caused my body to spasm as it did. The test results never revealed what the tissue originally was.

The tissue could have been a cancerous tumor. It could have been some leftover embryonic tissue. Frankly, I believe it was more likely to be leftover embryonic tissue. I base my opinion less on what my doctors said at the time, and more upon what happened later, what I have read, and differing opinions from other physicians. Either way, cancer or embryonic, the mass was there and caused havoc, and after surgery, it was gone.

Since I had not eaten or had anything to drink for several days, my digestive system had shut down and needed a restart. Working to get my system restarted was one of the reasons they kept me in the hospital. The process was slow and agonizing, as my stomach struggled to handle even the blandest of foods. Honestly, I had no idea gas could be that painful. No wonder babies cry when they have gas.

Another reason I was kept in the hospital was to watch for post-surgery infections. In fact, the night after my first surgery, I developed an elevated temperature, not quite enough of a fever to alarm the medical staff, but enough of a rise that my nursing staff grew concerned. The night nurse who was assigned to my room was amazing. Actually, all of the nurses were fantastic. Out of the hundreds of nurses I've met, there has been only one who was not fantastic.

The night shift nurses, at the time, tended to be what the locals called "gypsies." They were called so because they traveled from hospital to hospital all over the West, settling down in none of them. Staffing in some remote Western areas can be difficult to maintain, so nurses who were willing to move from town to town received substantial signing bonuses, housing stipends, the works. These nurses moved around for a great many different reasons, but most did it to pay off school loans quickly. All of these mobile nurses who worked with me were super nice and very good at what they did, but almost all of them worked nights.

The night nurse who took care of me after my major surgery was monitoring my temperature. It was inching up every hour that night. I was fortunate that I had the room all to myself. I recall the nursing staff discussing how they wanted to address the temperature rise. Should they use aspirin or maybe something else to start? They put a call in to the surgeon and waited for his orders. The night nurse chatted with me; most of the nursing staff did when they had time, and she asked if she could try something besides additional meds first.

As I mentioned, Flagstaff is up in the mountains, so most nights the temperature drops, and it drops quickly. Being late September, the temp was in the fifties or lower that night. She opened the window and closed my door. I felt the night air pour into the room immediately. The air did not feel cold at first due to my elevated temperature. A few hours later, the air began to feel cold, and my fever was gone. It's funny how old-fashioned remedies can still work.

Nurses have a rough job, and thank God for these compassionate, caring, and loving people, women and men, who take on the role. Nursing can be an incredibly thankless job. They see people, often at their worst. They are in a high-stress profession, where their action or inaction can be the difference between life and death. They are on point, the boots on the ground of the medical profession. I am grateful to everyone one of them.

Nurses are incredibly important to the care of all who are sick and hurting. A nurse's work can be gross and thankless, but they still do the work because they care. They are commissioned to care for us and for those we love. I am so thankful for the women, and men, who have chosen this profession.

May God bless you all!

How has a nurse impacted your life positively?

Have you thanked your nursing staff?

What led you to serving as a nurse?

Romans 15:1 (ESV): "We who are strong have an obligation to bear with the failings of the weak, and not to please ourselves."

Chapter 13

I was released from the hospital a few days later. My stay lasted six days. My temperature was stable, and my drainage was "clear" and not too heavy. Drainage was a byproduct of the surgery, and it was measured by how much gunk filled the bulb attached to the tubing snaked around inside my body. It was at this point, when the nursing staff showed us how to keep the bulb and tubing clean, that my wife named it my "Little Buddy."

I was always conscious of my Little Buddy. I had to be. One night, I accidentally caught the bulb on the hospital bed frame, and it gave the bulb and the tubing a solid tug, a tug that smarted quite a bit. After that tug, I never forgot to make sure the bulb and tubing were stowed in a safe place, such as a pajama pocket.

We had one last check-in with the surgeon and my nurse practitioner before I was discharged from the hospital. The medical staff was not quite sure what the necrotic tissue had been, as the results came back inconclusive. It was as dead as dead could be, basically. The plan, going forward, was to keep me on strong pain meds for a few weeks until my body had recovered from the surgery, and then we would see what developed. The human body is a complex organism, and we do not always get the answers we seek.

I was given a script for a very strong pain med and another for a prescription-strength heartburn reliever. My stomach was still experiencing severe gas pain several days after I had gone back on solid food. It took about ten days before my stomach was back to normal.

During this long hospital stay, several people from church came to visit, including my Sunday school class, my pastor, my friends, and my elders. I had a lot of visitors, all of them kind and gracious, not just to me, but also to the entire medical staff. By the end of my stay, the nursing staff was sad to see me go. I endeavored to be the best patient possible for them by being the most joyous person there. And I was successful.

My witness, or my sharing Jesus with people, is through two main avenues. I use words, spoken or written. But I also witness to others in how I behave toward them or treat them, as Jesus tells us in Matthew 5:16: "In the same way, let your light shine before others, so that they may see your good works and give glory to your Father who is in heaven."

While I was in the hospital, I made a conscious choice, no matter how awful I felt or how much pain I was in, that I would be content and would let my light shine. As the Apostle Paul wrote in Philippians 4:1–13 (ESV): "Not that I am speaking of being in need, for I have learned in whatever situation I am to be content. I know how to be brought low, and I know how to abound. In any and every circumstance, I have learned the secret of facing plenty and hunger, abundance and need. I can do all things through Him who strengthens me."

Learning how to be content in any given situation is a skill I continue to work on. Contentment is not happiness. It is an entirely different thing from happiness. Happiness is temporary. It can be fleeting. For example, I was happy when I was able to eat and drink after surgery, but when the gas pain hit moments later, I was not happy anymore.

Contentment, however, has helped me to find joy (which is what Philippians is all about). I have come to believe that measuring everything by how happy I am is not realistic, satisfying, or necessarily biblical. Before my faith, what made me happy one day would be unsatisfying the next, so pursuing happiness was a maddening cycle. When I added in the fact that my circumstances were so often out of my control, focusing on "being happy" does not work for me. I was not happy about being in the hospital. I was not happy I had to have the emergency abdominal surgery. I was not happy about the pain. I was, however, able to accept the circumstances and be content in them.

How? How did I learn contentment? If I trust God with my eternal destination, shouldn't I trust Him with my life and my circumstances here? If He is truly in control, aren't my circumstances also in His hands? I found peace and contentment in this knowledge.

I was released and sent home with my wife and son. Back then, we lived in a second-floor apartment sitting above our complex's laundry room. Those stairs were a bit of a challenge for me post-surgery, which came as a bit of a shock. Before the surgery, I was hiking 15 miles at a time, up and down steep mountainous terrain, with a full pack of water on my back. After the surgery, those fifteen steps were my Mount Everest.

With Laura holding my arm, I was able to get to the top. I had to wait for a moment at the top, as I was breathless and dizzy. I was holding the railing in a death grip. After the dizziness settled, I entered my apartment, happy to be home after nearly a week in the hospital.

My convalescence at home went well. I received several visitors, and my recovery sped along. However, I do want to share some things. I have mentioned pain meds a lot. I did not have, nor do I have, issues with pain meds to this day. I do, however, understand why people develop an addiction to them. Other than morphine, I was able to keep the pain meds under control. I did this by cutting back on them as quickly as I could. I probably cut back too soon. I was not, however, totally addiction free.

About a week after I returned home, I had an appointment with my nurse practitioner. I thought this was going to be a checkup in which I could order a pain med refill. My schedule was pretty much set. I would take a single pill at 5 A.M., 1 P.M., and 9 P.M. This was half the suggested daily dosage. I had set this schedule as it worked quite well for me and helped me manage the pain and the meds.

My appointment was with the nurse practitioner at around 11 A.M., the tail end of my first pain med of the day. That morning I had taken my last one, so I needed a refill. I thought Jane would look me over, and then I would get a refill and be set to take my next med at 1 P.M. All would be well if things went according to my schedule.

As happens from time to time, doctors and nurse practitioners have patient emergencies and their schedules change at the last minute. Of course, on this day, my nurse practitioner had been called away to the hospital, but she would be back in the office around noon. I figured I might be a little late on the 1 P.M. pill, but fine, I could hack it. It would be a good test of my pain management.

Jane did get in at noon, but she did not see me until 12:30–12:45 P.M. or so. I was led back and we chatted for a while about my recovery, how I was feeling, how active I was—all the normal questions. Then she told me she was going to remove the tubing from my stomach. I am not sure what face I gave her—maybe sheer terror—but whatever my face conveyed, it was enough of an alarm that she was taken aback. She asked me if I had taken my pain meds that morning. I answered honestly that I had taken one at 5 A.M. and needed a refill. Looking at her watch, I could see her doing the quick math. It was nearly eight hours after my last pain med. She excused herself and scrambled, looking for any kind of pain med in her office. There were none.

We discussed the need to have the tubing removed, regardless of whether or not I had any pain meds. We decided together it would be better to "rip off the band-aid," almost literal in this case, and get the tubing out. The tubing had been in long enough already, and the longer we delayed, the more difficult it would be to remove. In preparation, Jane had me lie back on an examining table, and she told me exactly what she was about to do and what would happen. She was going to give a firm tug on the tube at first as the tubing coming out of my stomach would be "stuck" to the incision site and in places inside. The sharp tug would break it free, and then she would keep pulling until it was out. It was going to be painful and I needed to relax as much as possible.

Once the "stuck" pieces became unstuck (i.e., ripped free), the rest of the tube should slide out easily. She did warn me of two things: once she started she was not going to stop, no matter how much I complained, and it would take a minute or two to get all of the tubing out. There was quite a bit of it, a few feet.

I wish I had stayed in touch with her, as I would love to get her thoughts on what happened next. Jane braced herself, planting her feet next to the examination table. I grasped the side of the table. Jane asked me if I was ready. I nodded and gritted my teeth. She was strong, I'll give her that. Jane got a solid grip and gave a very firm tug, I felt the skin puckered around the tube tear a bit then the tubing began sliding out.

My breath was stuck in my throat. White knuckled, lying on the table, the tube came out inch by inch and I felt all of it. I cannot quite describe the feeling, nor will I describe what it looked like. About halfway through the procedure Jane started yelling at me, "Breathe, BREathe, BREATHE!"

I forced myself to breathe, and finally I felt the final bit of the hose come out. We both were panting a bit after the procedure was finished. She asked me, softly, if I was OK. All I could say was, "That was interesting." Again she laughed. I was given a few moments to catch my breath while she bandaged the small hole in my belly. Then I was told my pain meds would be waiting for me at my pharmacy, and to please take it easy. I stood shakily and waited a few moments to get my bearings.

The other event was related to the addiction I was fighting at the time. I had developed a one- to two-can-per-week habit of chewing tobacco over the years. During stressful times, it was 2.5 cans. While I was in the hospital, and after being home for a week or two, I had not had any chewing tobacco. Instead of taking the opportunity to quit the habit, I planned for my first solo excursion out of the apartment to secure a fresh can.

After being home for several days, Laura felt it was OK for me to be left alone, and honestly, I needed some alone time. I had had someone with me or by my side constantly for two weeks. Getting some alone time was necessary, and it was exciting for me. On my first day alone, I put a plan into action to get tobacco. I worked on going up and down the stairs on day one. Then I worked on walking around the courtyard of our complex and the stairs on day two. On day three, I decided to make the trek to the closest gas station to buy a can of chewing tobacco. Day three of my preparation had originally been a day to walk up and down the main road out in front of the complex, which was flat. The idea was to build up some strength. Instead, I decided to go for the tobacco.

The gas station was two-tenths of a mile from our apartment complex—too bloody far, actually. In my mind, the best part of my intended trip was that the gas station was downhill. It was a steep downhill, but downhill, nonetheless. Getting there would be fairly easy, and as long as I took my time, I should be OK for the climb back up the hill, and I would have the chew.

I had to scrounge around the apartment to find the $5.00 I needed. My wallet was empty, and I had not been to the bank in weeks. If I remember correctly, I had a pocketful of change and I could not find any cash. I couldn't ask for cash, either, as that would tip Laura off. I knew that Laura knew I chewed. We just didn't discuss it, and asking for cash would have raised questions I didn't want to answer at the time.

With $5.00 in coins in my pocket, I made the trek. Going downhill was easy, and I was able to get into the gas station, buy my brand of chew, and head back up the hill. However, I realized I was in trouble when I left the store. I had a hard time opening the heavy door to get out. The effort to open the door left me dizzy. My plan had been to put some chew in immediately, but I was too dizzy to do even that. I swayed on my feet for a while. I had to lean against the building for a few minutes until the dizziness stopped. One of the locals asked me if I was OK. I just nodded and mumbled, "Tired."

Once I got my head under control, I started walking up the hill in small, shuffling steps. I stopped three times going up the hill, waiting for the dizziness to pass each time. When I reached the top of the hill, I was layered in sweat. The temperature was in the low 70s, and my clothes were drenched. I was able to get back to the apartment, but the four-tenths of a mile round trip took nearly ninety minutes. Once I hit the apartment, I didn't open the chew; instead, I slept for hours after changing out of my sweat-stained clothes. But I got my chew.

Years later, I cannot believe how stupid I was, and for so long. I chewed tobacco on and off for years. I was finally able to quit using tobacco entirely, but it took a lot of work and a lot of prayer. I tell people there are some things you should just never see, and some things you should never try—tobacco is one of them. If you use tobacco, quit now. If you have never tried tobacco, don't. It's not worth it.

Addictions are powerful and require a lot of work and help to overcome. If you are struggling with addiction, please find help; it can be beaten.

Do you struggle with an addiction?

Do you need help in overcoming an addiction?

Do you know someone who is struggling with addiction? Opioids? Porn? Tobacco? Alcohol?

1 Corinthians 10:13 (ESV): "No temptation has overtaken you that is not common to man. God is faithful, and He will not let you be tempted beyond your ability, but with the temptation He will also provide the way of escape, that you may be able to endure it."

Chapter 14

While convalescing, I started pushing myself and going on more and longer walks around the property and the surrounding part of town. Our apartment complex was just off the main street of Flagstaff, Milton Road, on the west side. This part of town is heavily populated with pine. It is also very hilly, so short walks were impactful. I planned on being back to work by Halloween. The company was planning for me to be back by then, and my recovery progressed well.

I was progressing well up until Friday, October 25th. The previous night, I started to feel pain in one of my testicles. The pain had probably been there for a while, and I just had not noticed, because everything else hurt so much more. Or the pain had been masked by the pain meds. By the end of October, I was off the pain meds entirely, and I was sticking with over-the-counter pain relievers.

Thursday night, the pain in my testicle was so bad that I opened up the medicine cabinet and grabbed one of my pain meds. It did not help dull the pain. So I thought applying heat might help. I grabbed a heating pad and stuffed it between my legs, positioned against the testicle. The heat did help.

My wife and I had been praying about the mass and what it had been, all while hoping the surgery had taken care of everything. That night, with the testicle pain, I recall praying that I wanted a clear signal. Had I pulled something in my groin, or was this something more severe?

God, please give me a sign.

When I awoke the next morning, I was alone in the apartment except for this grapefruit-sized swelling, which was my testicle. Overnight it had swelled up to the size of a grapefruit, or at least a large orange. It hurt terribly, and I had my sign. I called Laura, who called my doctor, who agreed to see me as soon as I could get there. I dressed very, very carefully. While I waited, I did a bunch of research on the internet, all of it kind of scary. All signs pointed toward testicular cancer.

For years, I had been terribly afraid of getting testicular cancer. I cannot explain why I had this fear, but it was there. This had started after watching *Brian's Song*, a wonderful TV movie from 1971 about Brian Piccolo and Gale Sayers' friendship during their time with the Chicago Bears. Slight spoiler: one of them develops testicular cancer.

In fact, I prayed specifically about not getting testicular cancer for years. The fear had abated some after my son was born. I remember having a strange thought one night, though. While I was praying for me, I also prayed that he would not get that cancer, either. Then this thought entered my mind during the prayer: if there was a choice between my son getting testicular cancer or me, which would I prefer? My answer was that I'd rather get the cancer myself than have to watch my son struggle with it. After thinking about it this way, the fear was mostly laid to rest.

And this Friday, here I was, a few weeks after his first birthday, with a testicle the literal size of a grapefruit, realizing I was probably going to face my biggest fear, and I would hear a cancer diagnosis that very day.

Walking around was difficult, especially with blue jeans on. No matter how I moved, the seam of my pants rubbed against that grapefruit. I had grabbed the loosest pair I owned, and still the denim rubbed against the swelling in my shorts. Laura called to say she was a few minutes away, so I made my way slowly down the steps and waited for her in the parking lot.

When she arrived, Laura pulled up by the sidewalk. I took one look at her and discovered she was white as a sheet. Laura had the car moving before I even closed the car door. Thinking ahead, I pulled the seam of my jeans downward when I sat down so it did not tighten up against my groin as it tended to do. The drive over to the doctor's office was quick and uneventful. I am sure Laura peppered me with questions. I do not remember.

We walked into the doctor's office together. My doctor's nurse led me back as soon as I walked in. She took my weight and my blood pressure. My weight was around 240. I'm a big guy, an inch or two over six feet and thick, as my mom used to say. After vitals were taken, the nurse led me to an examination room. My doctor quickly came in, asked me to describe what was going on, and then had me drop my pants. As soon as he saw my testicle, he winced.

After feeling around some and checking my prostate again, my doctor called over to the hospital. I needed to have an ultrasound test, and afterward would need to come back to his office to discuss our next steps. Laura and I drove over to the hospital. By this time, I was numb. I wanted to skip through all this crap and get to the obvious diagnosis, but I knew I'd have to go through these steps.

The wait at the hospital was short. An incredibly nice young woman was to be my ultrasound technician. She was a tad nervous, but she kept it clinical as she described what I needed to do. Disrobe, lie on my back, point my penis toward my belly button, and place a towel on top of my penis. Place another towel beneath my scrotum so it was pushed up and easier for her to run the scanning probe over it. I have to confess that when I first saw the probe, I flashed back to the invasive GI tract scan. My tech assured me this scan would not be invasive.

After following her directions to prep myself for her scan, she warned me of two things. One, the gel she was going to use was cold. And second, she would be as gentle as she could, but considering the condition of the testicle, running the probe over it would likely hurt. It did hurt, but just not too badly. After completing her test, she handed me another fresh towel, which she had somehow warmed up, to clean myself with, and then I was sent on. This young lady was amazing, and her ability to keep an uncomfortable situation so professional, and yet nice, helped me mentally.

It was during this scan I started praying a certain way, which became my common practice during these situations. Lying there while she ran the probe over me, I wanted to pray, but I couldn't think of any words to pray. I was drawing a complete blank. So I started praying the Lord's Prayer: "Our Father which art in heaven, Hallowed be thy name. Thy kingdom come, Thy will be done in earth, as it is in heaven. Give us this day our daily bread. And forgive us our debts, as we forgive our debtors. And lead us not into temptation, but deliver us from evil. For thine is the kingdom, and the power, and the glory, for ever. Amen" (Matthew 6:9–13 KJV).

I prayed the Lord's Prayer over and over again until the scan was complete. I'm not much on ritual (this is a preference of mine, and not a dogmatic statement), and I realize that saying the Lord's Prayer over and over again like a mantra is awfully ritualistic. I just did not have any other words to pray. The Lord's Prayer helped me have words so I could continue to connect with my Lord and my God.

After the scan, we headed over to the doctor's office. We did wait for a while, as the doctor was awaiting the radiology results. Eventually I was called back. Laura stayed in the waiting room. My general practitioner was waiting for me. He spoke quickly and asked if it would be OK if another doctor saw me. I gave him permission, and he left.

A few minutes later a very tall, good-looking, red-headed doctor walked in and introduced himself. He was a urologist from

Cottonwood who was visiting my GP as he and his family made their way to a weekend getaway in Vegas. He asked me a lot of questions, including about my history and recent health events.

After listening to me for a bit, he had me lie down on my back, and then he examined me head to toe, including both testicles. When the exam was finished, he had me sit up then began to share his background. He was a former department chair at a very large university in the Midwest, had studied under the physician who developed the protocol to fight testicular cancer, and had worked with more testicular cancer cases then he cared to mention.

This doctor, my urologist, gave it to me straight. The scan had been inconclusive at first pass, and the radiologist was going through the scan again. My urologist gave me his diagnosis based upon what he had felt. I likely had a mix of embryonal carcinoma and other germ cells. He even gave me a percentage of the cancerous mix, which turned out to be correct.

Embryonal carcinoma is a germ cell tumor that can occur in the testes as well as in the ovaries. They are distinct from other types of tumors because they are trying to "evolve" into their next stage of development (http://library.med.utah.edu/WebPath/MALEHTML/MALE092.html).

As my urologist pointed out to me, I was almost 100% average when it came to testicular cancer patients. I was 31 and the average age of testicular cancer patients is 31. My cancer appeared to be a mix of embryonal and other germ cells, which is typical of about 90% of testicular cancer cases (see *Sternberg's Diagnostic Pathology,* 5th Edition).

My urologist gave the news to me bluntly. The testicle in question would be removed. I would be given time to recover, and then an aggressive form of chemo and possibly radiation would be administered. The chemo would "kick my ass," and life would be hell for a few months, and then I would get better and I would be OK.

He then asked if I had any questions. I was still pretty numb, so I could not think of any. Then he noticed the ring on my finger and asked me if I was married and if my wife was with me. I said yes she was; she was out in the waiting room. He shook his head and berated himself. He had me go out to the waiting room and get her.

I left the examination room, went around the corner to the hallway, and opened the door to the waiting area. Laura anxiously looked up at me. I waved her to come back. She got up hurriedly and came back. Our son stayed with the nurse and office manager. My urologist was waiting for us.

Laura stood next to me when I sat back down on the exam table. She was holding my hand. The doctor then detailed everything he had found, what the next steps were, what it would be like, and what the expected results would be. Laura listened carefully and waited until he had finished.

"Do you have any questions?" he asked.

"Yes, will we be able to have more children?" Her voice was stressed, but there was no quiver in it, only a firm resolve.

The doctor thought for a moment and then asked if we had children today. We told him about our one-year-old our son. He nodded again and then said, "No, after the surgery, the chemo, and the radiation, you won't be able to have more children. I assume you want more?"

She nodded affirmatively. My urologist talked about artificial insemination and suggested we contact a sperm bank down in Phoenix that could help us prepare for the eventuality. Laura and the urologist chatted in a bit more detail about the surgery, the recovery period, and the potential complications. Laura was detailed and thorough in her questioning. Once we were through with the questions, my urologist confirmed that his nurse would schedule the surgery and get me set up with an oncologist.

Chapter 14

When we left the doctor's office, it was in the afternoon and we were both exhausted, although the hardest part of the day was yet to come.

I had to call back home and tell everyone the diagnosis: testicular cancer with a preliminary stage 3 evaluation. The assumption was the necrotic tissue was a metastasis of the cancer, and without further tests and scans, it would be likely I had cancer in some lymph nodes between the testicle and where the original necrotic tissue was found. My urologist did note that he had not felt any other lumps, but another scan would tell the tale. We all agreed that it would be prudent to assume the worst case scenario.

On the drive home, I tried calling my mom first. I figured she would be the best option. She didn't answer, so I left a brief message asking her to call back. After dropping me off, Laura left with our son to buy him a costume. The church was having a Halloween party that night and we planned on going. Very early on, even with the diagnosis, we decided to not disrupt our son's life, or our own, as much as possible.

I did call and talk to Pastor Bill. He was in California visiting his home. He listened attentively, asked when the surgery would be and when I would see the oncologist, basically making sure we had all of our bases covered. Then he assured us we would be in his prayers. We went to the Halloween party that night, but we waited until Sunday morning to tell our small group and the church.

On Sunday I shared the news. I cried for the second time post-diagnosis as I shared. I tried to be as specific as I could, and as everyone asked me what they could do, I simply asked them to pray. Keep it simple, I thought—simple prayer asking for healing, strength, wisdom, and guidance for my doctors.

Simple prayer. It's amazing to think of our prayers as simple. After all, praying is speaking to and being heard by the Creator. He hears all of our prayers. Prayer is such a simple act of faith, yet in our prayer we are acknowledging Him as our Lord, our God, and our

Savior, and He listens to us. Regardless of how old we are—child, adult, or senior citizen—He listens to us all.

I asked for prayer as I remembered what James taught us. In James 5:14–15 (ESV): "Is anyone among you sick? Let him call for the elders of the church, and let them pray over him, anointing him with oil in the name of the Lord. And the prayer of faith will save the one who is sick, and the Lord will raise him up. And if he has committed sins, he will be forgiven."

I understood I was asking for complete healing, and God could say, "No." I was willing to accept His answer, as it's the last part of this verse that speaks loudest to me. God can heal us, and He often does. Sometimes, as so many of us have experienced, He doesn't heal us, but when we approach Him in faith, He will always forgive.

Do you need healing? Do you want to be made well?

Has God ever told you No? What happened afterward?

Are you waiting on God to answer a prayer now? Who can pray with you during this time?

1 John 1:9 (ESV): "If we confess our sins, he is faithful and just to forgive us our sins and to cleanse us from all unrighteousness."

Chapter 15

The day of my cancer diagnosis, I had left my parents a message to call me back. Mom finally called back after Laura and our son got back from shopping. We had a few hours before we had to leave for the Halloween party at church. I must have had a tone in my voice when I left the message, as she was on high alert when she called me. It was a tough conversation, but it was not the toughest I would have that night.

After telling her everything about the diagnosis and the treatment plan, she said I needed to tell my father. Up to that moment, I had not considered that I would be the one to tell him. I was not looking forward to this. When Dad got on the phone, he definitely knew something was very wrong, and he asked me right away what was wrong.

I told him, "I have cancer."

He asked, "What kind?"

I informed him rather calmly, "I have testicular cancer."

He took a deep breath, and then my tough-as-nails dad completely lost it emotionally.

My father lost all semblance of control, of aloofness, of emotional distance. This tough, difficult man cried like a blubbering baby, insisting we move home, insisting that Indiana University (IU) had the best hospital and doctors for cancer. He was insisting that I could stay at home and he would drive me to my treatments every day. Then he told me he loved me.

This outburst was something I was not prepared for, nor was I equipped to handle it. I cried right along with him. Years of frustration, pain, fear, and doubt were washed away with those tears. As a parent, I have made it my primary goal for those I love to know unequivocally that I love them. I want them to understand and feel secure in my love. This is the kind of love that my Father in heaven has for me and for you. My friend, make sure those you love know it, and assure them that your love is unassailable.

After getting myself under some semblance of control, I assured Dad that my doctors were thorough, my urologist had worked with the doctors at IU, and we were going to undergo the treatments in Arizona. I did agree that if things went poorly, we would consider a move back home. Much later on, my mom shared with me that one of Dad's classmates had had the same cancer back in the '50s. His classmate must have had an advanced and aggressive form, as his treatment was radical and severe. They had literally cut him in half. He did not survive.

His classmate's cancer was well before the life-saving work of Dr. Lawrence Einhorn, his great team, and many other researchers and physicians around the globe who developed the protocol for testicular cancer. Before their work, the mortality rate, the death rate, for testicular cancer was 90% in the first year after diagnosis.

Today the survival rate for five years or longer is 95% (https://www.cancer.net/cancer-types/testicular-cancer/statistics).

After the Halloween party, we came home and our caller ID box was blinking, indicating a call and a voicemail. This was 2002, well before cell phones were ubiquitous. If we wanted to know who was calling us, we used to have to have these little boxes attached to our phone lines. These boxes would show a phone number and sometimes the name of the person calling. If you missed the call, or were not home, the caller ID box would flash a red or green light, depending on model. At the time, they were a crazy cool invention, and they helped screen unwanted calls.

Our caller ID box was flashing. I checked the box and saw that my grandfather had called six times. He had also left multiple voicemails. I had not called to tell him, but I let Mom do this. His last voicemail was the most moving; he simply said, "Call me back; I just want to hear your voice." Even though it was late back in Indiana, I called and we chatted for a few minutes, and then we agreed to check in regularly. I called my grandfather every week after that, sometimes twice a week, without fail. We talked every week up until he passed on.

After a very long day, Laura put our son to bed, and then she went to bed herself. I told her I would be up for a while. She hugged me, kissed me, told me she loved me, and asked if I would be OK. Did I want her to stay up with me? I smiled and said no. Laura was so tired she was swaying on her feet in exhaustion.

After the two of them went to bed, I turned the TV on for a few minutes, tried to find something to watch, and then switched it off. Tiredly I got to my feet, grabbed my Bible, my journal, and a candle. I went into the main bathroom and shut the door, locking it behind me. I drew a hot bath. My groin was hurting a bit, so I settled into the water to ease the pain.

In my journal, I wrote out my thoughts of the day and wrote several short prayers. Then I started reading my Bible. I believe I was in the book of Luke and read several chapters. The room was dark except for the single candle burning. The candle was on the floor, so I had enough light to read and write by. After a bit, my head clear of the day's worry, I laid my journal and my Bible aside and closed my eyes.

I began to pray. My prayers this night became a running monologue. I do not recall all of my words, but the overall message came down to this: I trust You, Lord, with my eternal salvation; I trust You with my life; I will trust You in this. It was as fervent a prayer as I could muster. I asked for healing, but I told Him I would accept what might come. And as I prayed, I felt a gathering Presence filling the room until I knew I was no longer alone.

As I prayed, a bright light began to seep through my closed eyelids. As a kid, have you ever closed your eyes and turned toward the morning sun? I used to do this quite often, feeling the warmth on my face. I especially enjoyed doing this in winter. Regardless of time of year, on a clear day, the sun is so bright it can pierce through your closed eyelids.

This night, the Light was similar to facing the sun, only this was much brighter. And this Light did not burn. Through my closed eyes, the Light was bright, golden, almost physical, yet somehow soft. I could sense the Light all around me. Not believing it, or thinking maybe the candle was producing a huge flame somehow, I cracked open my right eye. The Light was surrounding me completely. Its Source seemed to be high up, near the bathroom entrance. The candle was small and inconsequential in this Light. I could barely discern its flame.

Remembering scripture, and how people cannot look upon God and live, I shut my eyes again, and I simply stayed still, listening. With the Light came a peace that I cannot even begin to explain. In that moment, it was made clear to me that the cancer would not be taken away, but it would not kill me. What I was about to go through was part of His plan, and it would be for His glory. And the peace I received allowed me to willingly accept my cancer.

After a time, the Light dissipated and the room went dark, except for the small flame of the candle. This Presence shook me to my core. I have spoken of this only a few times, as it's not something I can speak about unemotionally, or even well. I wish I could say the rest of my cancer experience was calm and peaceful; it wasn't. I am not a super Christian. I wish I were, but I am a sinner, saved by the grace of Jesus Christ.

In our faith, amongst followers of Christ, people have hoped and prayed for something to happen to them like what happened to me that night. I don't know why God blessed me with His Presence. I don't know why others who have served God so wonderfully, and for many years, and with such steadfastness, have never experienced what I had experienced. Regardless of why, this event did happen, and I can do nothing but love the Lord. He is as real to me as my wife or my children.

The Psalms are a fantastic book of the Bible, and I recommend that believers and non-believers read them, especially those who, like me back then, are facing cancer, pain, disappointment, strife, or fear. And like me today, it is an amazing book of rejoicing for those who trust in Him and find joy in His Word.

My favorite Psalm is 116, I Love the Lord. Please read this and see if you can understand why it is so important to me:

Psalm 116 (ESV):

I love the Lord, because he has heard my voice and my pleas
    for mercy.
Because he inclined his ear to me, therefore I will call on him
    as long as I live.
The snares of death encompassed me; the pangs of Sheol laid
    hold on me; I suffered distress and anguish.
Then I called on the name of the Lord: "O Lord, I pray, deliver
    my soul!"

Gracious is the Lord, and righteous; our God is merciful.
The Lord preserves the simple; when I was brought low, he
    saved me.
Return, O my soul, to your rest; for the Lord has dealt
    bountifully with you.

For you have delivered my soul from death, my eyes from
    tears, my feet from stumbling;

I will walk before the Lord in the land of the living.

I believed, even when I spoke: "I am greatly afflicted";
I said in my alarm, "All mankind are liars."

What shall I render to the Lord for all his benefits to me?
I will lift up the cup of salvation and call on the name
 of the Lord,
I will pay my vows to the Lord in the presence of
 all his people.

Precious in the sight of the Lord is the death of his saints.
O Lord, I am your servant; I am your servant, the son of
 your maidservant.
You have loosed my bonds.
I will offer to you the sacrifice of thanksgiving and call on the
 name of the Lord.
I will pay my vows to the Lord in the presence of all his
 people, in the courts of the house of the Lord, in your
 midst, O Jerusalem.
Praise the Lord!

Chapter 16

Over the next couple of days post-diagnosis, I spent a great deal of time calling friends and family, making sure I had as many people and churches praying for me as possible. Prayer was a key component of our cancer battle strategy. In fact, I know there was a church as far away as Sweden that was praying for me. (Thank you Jenny H!)

My local church lined up childcare, food, and transportation to wherever we needed. The church, and I mean the entire body of Christ, is at its best when it's mobilized to do three things: sharing the Gospel, developing believers (sanctification), and helping those in need. No politics (and by politics, I mean leave your ideology at home—right, left, or other), no gossip, nothing extra, just people following Christ. The body of Christ surrounded me and my family in prayer and in physical action, as my favorite pastor says, "It's where the rubber meets the road."

Besides making all of those calls, another part of our strategy was to study up on the enemy. I read up on my cancer and what to expect. A statistic I encountered over and over again was that people are more afraid of the treatment than of the cancer itself. Knowledge helps dispel fear, and I wanted to learn as much as I could. Laura, for her part, studied nutrition as it relates to fighting cancer and recovery. She read that the chemotherapy would be so strong that I would need two meals at each sitting. One meal I would eat and throw up, and the second, high in nutrition, I could hopefully keep down.

Laura also became an authority on which vitamins, minerals, and supplements she could add to my diet that would not only help my body cope with the chemo, but would also help my body fight the cancer inside it. And, God love her, she also studied up on what, if anything, could prevent me from becoming sterile. More than anyone else, Laura developed the battle plan for my cancer. The doctors were there to help us in the fight, but the battle plan was hers.

My urologist's office called and let me know my surgery would be on Thursday morning, October 31st, Halloween. They moved the surgery out as far as they dared, as I was still resting up and recovering from my exploratory abdominal surgery. A few days' extra rest would be helpful. I was given my pre-surgery instructions, and I prayed often.

The night before my second surgery, I was cut off from any food or liquids. I think the cutoff time was 11 P.M. I remember thinking how much I had hated being so dry before my first surgery, so I drank a large glass of water right before 11 P.M. Honestly, I may have had two large glasses. My goal was to not feel so parched after surgery.

Laura and I got up early the next day, as the surgery was scheduled to put me first in line. I prefer early procedures and early surgeries. I prefer the early start so I do not have to wait around in the morning for procedures or surgeries.

The pre-op was simple and uneventful, save for one incredibly odd request one of the nurses asked me to do. The OR nurse who would be assisting my urologist, who would be performing the surgery, introduced herself. In the pre-op room, I was in my gown and nothing else, trying to not be nervous about what was to occur. The nurse smiled and told me that she was there to make sure I was ready and to confirm why I was there. She then asked me to tell her why I was there.

I explained I was there for an inguinal orchiectomy. She blinked a few times and said, "I wasn't expecting that, the correct medical terminology. People usually say something more crude." Then she reached into her pocket, pulled out a blue felt tip marker, and handed it to me.

I accepted the marker, holding it in front of me quizzically. I wanted to laugh as I found this to be somewhat comical, being handed a felt tip marker in pre-op. My first thought was that she was handing the marker to me for my son, who was in the room with us. Looking at the marker, and then back to the nurse, I asked her, "What am I supposed to do with this?

She said, "Write an X on it," pointing toward my groin. "Write an X on the testicle that is being removed. We don't want the doctor to remove the wrong one."

My gut lurched and I nearly threw up. There was something truly horrifying in her statement. Honestly, if the doctor could not tell the difference between the two the way they were, then I was in serious trouble. One was still the size of a grapefruit, after all. Taking no chances, though, I "X"ed the correct testicle with the marker. I felt like throwing up again when I handed the marker back. I still feel a chill every time I think about the marker conversation. After the nurse left with her marker, the anesthesiologists came in and met with me. They were very nice. They discussed what they were going to do and then put me to sleep quickly.

When I was a teenager, we had what had to be the dumbest black Labrador retriever in the history of black lab dogs. He was also the most loving dog ever. His heart was a lot bigger than his minuscule brain. His name was Herbie, named not after the VW car, but for some unknown reason, after President Herbert Hoover.

My paternal grandmother had a few acres of land out in the country. On her property she had a fishing pond that also doubled as a swimming hole. Often my dad, my brother, and I would go fishing together. And if it was hot enough, my brother and I would go swimming in the pond.

From time to time we would take the dog with us. Mom hated that dog, and truly he was a pain. He dug up all of her flower beds, making him the bane of her existence. He was not very useful. If we took him hunting, he would eat, or try to eat, whatever we successfully shot. And he was too fast, always arriving before we could get there. We tried obedience training, but it did not stick.

Fishing was a nightmare with Herb. The dog would splash around wherever we threw our lines in, zeroing in on the bobber, thinking we were playing a game of catch or something. With Herb along, we almost never caught anything. But some days it was better to have him with us and give Mom a break. That dog really loved her.

When we did catch a fish, it was a race to get it off the line before the dog grabbed it and took off. Herb weighed around 75 pounds, and he would bend the fishing pole so severely, it nearly broke every time he grabbed a fish and took off. Luckily, he never hooked himself.

On one of our fishing trips, Herb had been particularly aggressive with me and my fishing pole, so I gave up and decided to go for a swim. Dad was up at Grandma's house. My brother was on the bank fishing. Stripped down to my swim trunks, I jumped into the cold water from off the pier and began swimming. After surfacing, I heard a loud splash. Herb had jumped in and swam toward me as fast as he could.

I did not think much of it. In fact, I thought it might be fun to grab his collar and have him pull me around the pond. Instead, the dumb thing swam right up to me and then tried to climb on my back. All of his weight hit me like a ton of bricks in the water. I was not ready for it and was pushed under. I tried to swim down away from him, but I panicked. My lungs filled with water and I thought how stupid, drowning by dog.

Then I heard another big splash, and my brother picked up Herb, throwing him off me. Then he grabbed me and pulled me onto land. I was still conscious, but my chest felt full and weighted. All of that water was sitting in my lungs. My brother, Paul, turned me on my side and all of the water came pouring out. Someone once told me drowning was peaceful; well, they are full of it. Drowning was not peaceful for me. I could feel the weight of the water in my chest, I could not breathe, and my brain felt as if it were on fire.

When I awoke from my surgery on Halloween, I woke up feeling heavy. My eyelids felt as if someone had placed weights on them. My chest felt full and heavy. Barely awake, coming slowly out of the anesthesia, I realized I could not breathe. I cracked an eye open and could see, through fuzzy vision, a nurse tending to another patient across the room from me. I tried raising my hand to signal him. I tried to speak, but my lungs pushed water up, but no air. I closed my eyes again and prayed. I must have made some noise because I heard the nurse yell an expletive, the sound of him rushing over, his hands grabbing me, and then I was turned on my side. And then a massive gush of fluid flew out of my mouth and nose.

Later on, my oncologist was looking at an x-ray taken of my chest right after I woke up from that surgery. The x-ray appeared to show I had an advanced case of pneumonia, as there was an enormous amount of fluid in my lungs. My oncologist started to chastise me and then I told her, "That's fluid from my stomach." She then grabbed the second x-ray, which was taken an hour after the first one. The second x-ray and the timestamp showed my lungs had mostly cleared up an hour or two later. What we believe happened was a pure accident. I bit down on the breathing tube when it was removed from my esophagus. By biting down, I caused a suction to occur, which pulled everything in my stomach up, out, and then down into my lungs. It was an accident, and thankfully the OR nurse, Mike, was alert and he saved my life. I'm grateful to him and to my brother, two men who saved me from drowning—one by dog, one in post-op.

Who has made a difference in your life? A teacher, a doctor, a sibling, a grandparent?

How and why did they make such a difference?

How has God made a difference in your life?

Psalm 116:3-4 (ESV): "The snares of death encompassed me; the pangs of Sheol laid hold on me; I suffered distress and anguish. Then I called on the name of the Lord: "O Lord, I pray, deliver my soul!"

Mathew 14:30 (ESV): "But when he saw the wind, he was afraid, and beginning to sink he cried out, 'Lord, save me.'"

Chapter 17

After the near drowning accident, I was moved to a room upstairs in the hospital. Originally, my inguinal orchiectomy was planned to be outpatient, but with the accident, the hospital staff wanted to keep an eye on me overnight. They also became very strict. The hospitals in the area are all wonderful institutions, staffed by excellent doctors and nurses, and with the accident they were not going to take any more chances with me.

My urologist left immediately after surgery to go to a Rascal Flatts concert. He could not check on me in person. He was with his family several hours away. I do recall overhearing him on more than one call, expressing his extreme displeasure with the accident. He checked on me regularly while I was in the hospital, as did my general practitioner. I made Halloween interesting for them.

While in my room, my groin started to ache a bit. It was not as bad as carrying around the grapefruit testicle, but it was enough that I finally asked about pain meds. They offered me morphine, which I declined, so I was given a lower-grade pain med that helped. I also asked about an ice pack. My urologist said icing my groin down would help with the discomfort.

Because the hospital and staff were taking no chances with me, I was not allowed to have an ice pack because the doctor had not ordered one. The hospital would not dispense an ice pack without a signed order, so no written order, no ice pack. It was unlikely that I would expire from an ice pack, but they were not going to take a single chance with me. On all of my future surgeries, I recounted the near-drowning experience, and every medical professional reacts in the same way: shock, and sticking to only written orders.

Once released again, I focused on recovery, walking a few miles each day and getting used to having only one testicle, which surprisingly took a few days. Having only one testicle threw my gait and my balance off. I also became very protective of the remaining one. I still am. My family and I own a horse and are quite active. I always wear a cup whenever I'm around horses. I take no chances in protection.

My doctors cautioned me to take it easy physically. Apparently, if I put too much pressure on my groin from working out, or hiking too much, or just walking too far, I could cause a tear in my inguinal wall that would cause internal bleeding, and it would be nasty. I reduced my walking down to just a mile each day. We wanted me to be in the best physical shape possible. Laura and I had been reading that the better my physical condition when I started chemo, the better I would be able to handle it. My daily exercise was a part of Laura's battle plan.

Physically, I was improving quickly. I did not feel that I had cancer. I would not have been able to hike fifteen miles, but I was feeling a whole lot better. At my last medical check-in, my weight was down to 219 pounds. I felt strong for the first time in months. I vowed to myself that I would tackle chemo head on.

Our first appointment with our oncologist came up. The best oncologist in the state of Arizona at the time happened to work in Sedona. We agreed with my urologist that the best course of action for me was to drive down to Sedona regularly. If I needed people to drive me, our church stood by to chauffeur me up and down the mountain.

The trip from Flagstaff to Sedona is roughly a 30-mile drive to the south by the main route, 89A. It is farther if the interstate is taken. There is a shorter mileage route, called Schnebly Hill Road—

shorter in a mileage sense. In the time sense, it takes several hours, as the route is a high-clearance road, one lane, with severe drop-offs. We almost always drove State Route 89A whenever we visited Sedona.

State Route 89A is an incredibly beautiful drive. The road curls through deep forest, and it has numerous switchbacks down the side of the mountain into Oak Creek Canyon, and on to Sedona, through town, and farther on into the Red Rock country. Sedona, Oak Creek Canyon, Flagstaff, and the Grand Canyon are some of our favorite places to visit. We loved living there and hope to do so again some day.

Our oncologist's Sedona office overlooks the Red Rock country. I have seen many oncology units over the years, and most of the units work at having a healing atmosphere, but not all of them are as aesthetically pleasing. At one particular unit that I have visited, all of the treatment chairs were lined up in an arc, all facing a central point in the unit, a single TV. The Sedona oncology unit had chairs broken into groups of four or five, all facing outward toward a series of large glass windows that overlooked one of the red rock mesas. Taking chemo while watching a TV or looking out at God's Creation? I'll choose looking outside every time.

Our first visit to oncology was thorough. We went through my personal history, my case history, and the protocol. My protocol was going to be a 12-week course of three different types of chemo drugs. My oncologist made sure I met with her entire nursing staff. Everyone was so caring, so loving, that we knew we were with the right medical staff. We brought our son with us, who was loved by everyone there, including the other patients.

My oncologist was tops in her field, which meant she got all of the difficult patients. By "difficult," I mean the types of patients who were given a two percent chance of survival. Here I was with my young beautiful wife, our incredibly adorable son, and a cancer that was curable. We were a hit. The nurses gobbled up the minutes they spent with our son, and they assured us that my being in peak physical condition, and having a tough wife and a son to fight for, I would make it through.

My oncologist ordered some additional tests. She wanted to make sure that I did not have any additional tumors, so I was set up for a full body scan on my November birthday. My chemo would start shortly after the CT scan results came back. The chemo would be in four rounds of three weeks each, for a total of twelve weeks. Each round would consist of etoposide, cisplatin, and bleomycin. If I remember correctly, the first week would be five straight days of etoposide and cisplatin, and then the bleo would be administered once during the first week or early on the second week. Radiation treatment was not initially within the plan, but it was held out if it became necessary.

The other two weeks of each three-week round would be rest, observation, blood tests, and if needed, an immune booster. The drugs would adversely affect my immune system, and if my bloodwork came back showing that my immune system was compromised or too low, then the oncologist would likely administer an immune booster. After learning about my personal treatment protocol and scheduling my CT scan, we left and headed back up the mountain toward home. We were as well educated and prepared as we could be. We knew the treatments were going to be rough, just not how rough it eventually became.

We had promised all of our friends and family that we would update them on the treatment plan once we were finished. Cell phone coverage between Sedona and Flagstaff was not the best, so I waited until we drove into the city before calling Pastor Bill. Pastor had asked me to call him once we were back. I did and outlined the protocol. He said, "You know they are trying to kill you, right? With that much chemo, they are going to get as close to it as they can, anyway."

It was not until Pastor said this that I realized how rough it might be. I am a firm believer in being pragmatic and truthful. It is the best way for me to prepare for whatever is to come.

What is the most daunting task you have ever faced?

How did you plan for the task or activity?

How did God support you in your task?

Joshua 1:9 (ESV): "Be strong and courageous; do not be frightened or dismayed, for the Lord your God is with you wherever you go."

Chapter 18

Before the orchiectomy surgery, and before chemo began, we needed to take care of a little matter of banking my sperm. Laura was adamant about having another child. I was not thrilled about the whole banking idea, especially having to drive down to Phoenix so I could provide a sample of my sperm. We did fight over this idea quite a bit, but she won out. Laura was the seventh child out of seven total kids. She came from a large family. Laura did not want our son to be an only child. While adoption was and is absolutely a viable option, Laura wanted to try the artificial insemination route first, or at least to have the option.

Our insurance at the time was decent, so the sperm bank tests were covered. All we had to pay for was storage. We drove down to Phoenix, about two hours away, and after hunting a bit, we found the place tucked away amongst other medical offices. I found the sperm bank experience to be incredibly odd. I was not so much embarrassed at being there as I was depressed about the need to be there, and the prospect of being sterile. The oddness of it all came from the obviousness of what I was there to do. I kept thinking everyone knows I am here to masturbate. How odd is that?

At our appointment, we talked through my circumstances with a doctor, and then we were ushered into a lab located at the back of the offices. In the lab we met a tech who handed me a cup and showed me to a dark room with a leather chair. Next to the chair was a table with a bunch of material that was there to aid me in my endeavor. Afterward, the tech asked me privately if I thought he needed to get new porn. How do you answer that question? Well, yes, the porn you have expired last fall. Do not misunderstand; I recommend banking sperm. As odd as it was for me, it was a necessity based upon the directions from my doctors.

The tech analyzed the sample I had provided and said he would need another sample to ensure that what we banked would be efficacious. We scheduled another visit a few days later, with the strict stipulation I wasn't to ejaculate for a few days. I did not bother to tell the tech about how my groin was the size of a grapefruit and that staying celibate would not be a problem. Laura, through all of this process, was patient yet persistent. I, however, started to worry about whether I would be able to perform well in the bedroom department when I would have only one testicle. My urologist told me my body would adjust, and he was right. It was during this time between diagnosis and surgery where I struggled mightily with the concern of having only one testicle. The impending reality of having just one really bothered me. And on the heels of the thought came the next one: would having only one testicle make me less of a man?

The answer, of course, is no, emphatically no. Biologically and fundamentally, I am a man. But such was my mental state and my own view of manhood. I had to work through it mentally. Having to go through the future child planning stage of banking my sperm made sure these thoughts were front and center.

While we were in the middle of this episode, the time between banking my sperm and my orchiectomy, my parents decided to fly out. They both needed to see me. Usually when we hosted people in Flagstaff, we went to the Grand Canyon, Lowell Observatory, Sunset Crater, Sedona, and other great places to sightsee and shop. For this visit, we did not do a whole lot. Mentally and physically, I was not up to doing much other than sitting around and chatting. Once the news broke back home in Indiana that I had cancer and was going through surgery and chemo, I started receiving cards and calls, far too numerous to count and impossible for me to list and to thank everyone by name. All I can say is how grateful I am to everyone who did reach out, who gave me words of encouragement and expressed their love so keenly. (A special thank you for the cards from Tabby and Janet—you know who you are!) I was receiving words, in due season, from all over the world, and they were all good!

Who are you supporting prayerfully now?

How can you broaden your prayer list?

If you need prayer now, who can you enlist to pray for you?

Proverbs 15:23 (ESV): "To make an apt answer is a joy to a man, and a word in season, how good it is!"

Chapter 19

After my orchiectomy, I was scheduled for another full body CT scan. The results would be used to determine and finalize my cancer stage. If I had any other tumors throughout my body, I would definitely be at stage three, although my bloodwork had come back indeterminate to additional tumors. The doctors expected to find an additional tumor or two in my lymph nodes. Lymph nodes are a key part of our body's immune system. Hundreds of these nodes are located throughout our bodies. They help our bodies fight infection and disease. With the necrotic tissue located behind my pancreas, the assumption was that the cancer had metastasized from my testicle up into my abdominal cavity via the lymph nodes. There should have been cancerous traces or small tumors in my lymph nodes. We hoped not, but it was a possibility we had to confirm or eliminate.

The CT scan itself was completely uneventful, although very lengthy. Fortunately, this time, I was able to drink the contrast dye the day before the scan, which is a whole lot better than having it delivered via the alien butt probe. The scan results showed nothing more than a few cold spots on my liver (normal) and a small, potentially cold nodule on my thyroid.

Cold nodules are areas of the thyroid that do not produce thyroid hormones. The thyroid is a butterfly-shaped organ that sits at the front of the neck beneath the Adam's apple. It converts iodine into a hormone called T4, which helps regulate metabolic rate, body temperature, and other things. The cold nodule on my thyroid would eventually need to be tested, but for now, we focused on the immediate need.

The scan, thankfully and—as one doctor said—almost miraculously, did not reveal any other tumors related to my testicular cancer. While the doctors would treat me as if the cancer had metastasized, post-surgery I was effectively free of any other detectable testicular cancer tumors in my body. This was great news and helped propel me into my chemo treatment with a positive attitude.

At the beginning of my chemo treatments, bloodwork became routine. Blood draws are simple and take just a few minutes. I had blood drawn from my hands, my arms, or pretty much anywhere a technician could find a "good vein." I have had my blood drawn hundreds of times over the past few decades. I can tell how good a phlebotomist is at the job just by how he or she touches my arm and looks for a vein.

At first, blood draws made me quite nervous. I worried about the potential results and what those results would mean for me. I consistently prayed for good results, and then after the draw, I would worry for hours or days as I awaited the results. My faith was regularly tested with all of these interminable waits. In hindsight, I worried needlessly. My advice is to accept a simple fact. Tests show us only what is going on or not going on. Ignorance can be deadly, and the tests confirm that all is well or show us what we absolutely need to know. Once we have the results, then we can rejoice or focus on how we need to address those results.

Jesus taught us in Matthew 6:24 (ESV): "Therefore do not be anxious about tomorrow, for tomorrow will be anxious for itself. Sufficient for the day, is its own trouble." I spent hours, days, and nights worrying about test results. The worry gained me nothing. It has taken me years of mental work, prayer, and confession to get the worry under some semblance of control. Recently, I had a series of tests run for a rare and severe blood-related condition, completely unrelated to my previous health issues. The results eventually pointed to something else, entirely different, simple, and definitely not severe. After nearly twenty years of tests and waiting for results, I can say I'm still working on the worry, but I am in a much better place now than when we waited on all those blood tests to come back at the beginning of my cancer treatment.

My bloodwork results were all positive early on—no tumor markers, white and red blood cell counts nominal—basically green lights across the board. I was perfectly healthy except for the cancer they had surgically removed. With this knowledge, my oncologist began my treatments.

She started off with a strong dose of chemo, with the intention of quickly upping my dosage. I am a big guy, and while I'm athletic, I am not a professional athlete, nor am I an amateur. I learned later that she had been working with oncologists at IU on my protocol and my treatment plan, all while coordinating with my urologist. As I look back, it still amazes me how deeply God was involved to bring these three amazing medical professionals together to treat me.

Have you ever had God answer a prayer directly and unquestionably? I have. Have you ever realized you were stuck in a bad spot, and an answer came from Him well before you even knew you needed to ask the question? I have. Throughout this experience, God was moving and putting people in place to treat me.

God answering prayer as soon as we begin to pray, or even before we know our needs, is biblical. In Isaiah 65:24, God tells us the day will come for all who are His: "Before they call, I will answer; while they are yet speaking, I will hear." And again in Daniel 9:23a: "At the beginning of your pleas for mercy, a word went out, and I have come to tell it to you, for you are greatly loved." With all of my pain up to this point and what was still to come, God had moved before

I even knew I needed to ask. Understand, at the time, I did not see any of these events as they were. It is only in hindsight that I can see how God was moving.

A prime example: I do not believe my urologist just happened to stop in for a visit with my GP, the very day, the very hour I needed him to take my case. It is no accident my GP was such a great doctor that he knew how and who to bring in to make sure I got the care I needed. It was no accident that the top oncologist in Arizona worked with the very doctor who developed the cure for my cancer and a urologist who had worked directly with the same oncologist. There are no coincidences or accidents like these. I know God was surrounding me and continues to surround me with doctors and nurses who care for me as a person and work hard to keep me healthy.

Have you ever prayed with your doctor? A nurse? I have. It is a life-changing event, and it changes how you see them and how they see you. God puts people in our lives for us to serve and for them to serve us. There are no coincidences with a loving God. (A dear friend used to call them "God Incidences.")

The first day of chemo came. Other than the large chemo needle going into my right hand, it was pretty painless. That first stick in my hand was the first of forty-seven. I remember the number, as I counted them all. For various reasons, my wife, my oncologist, and I had chosen to not install a port. A port is a temporary medical device that allows doctors and nurses to plug in IVs in one spot instead of constantly needing to stick a needle in different parts of the body. I did not choose a port, as I did not want another procedure unless it became absolutely necessary. I still agree with my decision. I will say, though, that having that big chemo needle digging around in my hand as it looked for a good vein could get tedious.

My first week of chemo went well. After the first week of treatment, I felt bloated most of the time. The chemo came in large bags, filled with what looked like gallons of fluid. Each bag dripped into me over several hours. During each treatment, besides the chemo, I was given two drugs.

At the start of each chemo drip, I was given Benadryl. The drug did two things that were blessings to me. First, it would help me if I happened to have an allergic reaction to any of the three chemo drugs. Second, it put me to sleep. I actually slept through most of my chemo treatments. I tended to stare out the windows at the Red Rock Mesa, and I would imagine living there a hundred years earlier. I always fell asleep within a few minutes.

The second drug was given to me near the end of each day's treatment. This second drug was a loop diuretic. Basically, it made me urinate. After taking the drug, I had to pee a lot, nearly nonstop. I hated that drug—loathed it, in fact. After a nice Benadryl nap, I would wake up to the injection. Once the injection was in me, I would have to force myself awake and start getting myself up and out of the chair, no matter how tired I was or how poorly I felt. I had to get started so I could make it to the bathroom on time.

Imagine drinking a gallon of water right before bed and then waking up groggily a few hours later with a bladder holding all of that liquid and your body ready to release, or as I used to tell my nurses, ready to fire away. It was a similar sensation. If I did not start for the bathroom early enough, it was hit or miss as to whether I would make it on time. Then imagine after urinating for five minutes with an unabated stream, you trudged back to bed or to your couch, and as soon as you sat down, you had a full bladder again. This cycle kept repeating until the drug wore off.

Near the end of my first week of chemo, I figured out a better routine. Once I was awake and out of my chair, and after I had urinated for the first time, instead of going back to my chair, I would walk around the oncology unit, wheeling my IV with me the whole way. It made it simple as I could stop and pee after each circuit of the unit, plus it helped to wake me up. This circuit became an essential survival routine for me.

Make me pee, that is what the loop diuretic did. Its function was to get all of the chemo fluid out of me. Even with this fluid being drained out, I still felt bloated and full. I called it "water fat." I felt bloated for a few weeks. That is, until the weekend after my second cycle of chemo.

God answers prayers. He has told me No. He has told me Yes. He has told me Not Yet.

God answers prayers. Pray, have friends pray, have churches pray. Pray for each other. Prayer works. There is a pattern in scripture of confession first, and then making our requests known before God. This is why I am sharing the full passage from chapter 9 of Daniel. This passage is one of my favorites in scripture, and it is a quick picture of this pattern. Daniel begins chapter 9 praying for his nation of Israel, and as soon as he starts praying, God has already moved to answer.

Do you believe God answers prayer?

How do you prepare yourself to pray?

Do you pray with a plan like Daniel or do you let God lead you in your prayer?

Daniel 9:20–23 (ESV): "While I was speaking and praying, confessing my sin and the sin of my people Israel, and presenting my plea before the Lord my God for the holy hill of my God, while I was speaking in prayer, the man Gabriel, whom I had seen in the vision at the first, came to me in swift flight at the time of the evening sacrifice. He made me understand, speaking with me and saying, 'O Daniel, I have now come out to give you insight and understanding. At the beginning of your pleas for mercy a word went out, and I have come to tell it to you, for *you are greatly loved.* Therefore consider the word and understand the vision.'"

Chapter 20

While my surgeries and my chemotherapy were going on, I was technically employed, but I was on a medical leave of absence. My employer was fair to OK about my medical leave. Frankly, my wife believed they were awful, as they tended to send important forms such as continuing health coverage deadline documents at the last minute, or their reps would give us erroneous information about deadlines, forms, or coverage. Laura believed this was intentional, as they wanted us to make a mistake so they could save a buck. My personal opinion is that they were incompetent, although it would not shock me to discover they were intentionally misleading.

When we first started having to fill out all of the necessary forms (an endless tidal wave of paper back then—electronic, for the most part, today), Laura took a crash course in how to read, understand, and correctly fill out these forms. Without her, we would have ended up in a very difficult financial place. Do not misunderstand; we still owed a lot of money for my medical care, but insurance covered a very large portion. Without Laura filling everything out and tracking all the deadlines, we would have gone bankrupt.

Our oncologist and the northern Arizona medical community were outstanding. All of them had fantastic advisors who walked us through their understanding of our insurance, our financial requirements, and our own needs, and they helped us put plans together so all we had to do was focus on the treatments and healing. Regardless of the financial situation, insurance situation, or lack thereof, the communities in which we all live have people dedicated to helping patients figure out the financial end of their situation. Most of them are social workers, who provide an invaluable service. Whenever we have had to set up payment schedules, whether it is a hospital or a doctor's office, all of them have been more than happy to work with us and to make it as easy as possible.

In fighting cancer, I had enough to worry about, and with my wife focusing on the paperwork, the long term disability (LTD) insurance, COBRA, and the forms, I was able to put all of it aside and zero in on fighting the disease, and to a certain extent, the chemotherapy. Thankfully, once my company's short term disability ran out, I had signed up for the long term disability at 60% of my pay. This enabled us to maintain an income, pay bills, and put gas in the tank of the car, which removed a mental burden.

If you have access to long term disability for yourself or for a loved one, I highly recommend it. I would also recommend looking into Long Term Care (LTC) insurance, the sooner the better. I can attest that having the financial end tied up eliminates a lot of worry for most people. I trust the Lord, and do so for everything. I do not believe that investing a few dollars into LTD or LTC is foolish or demonstrates lack of trust in God. Not everyone can afford these programs, but there are always options. We have to keep looking, and asking until we find the help we need.

A lot of scripture is just plain common sense, or what used to be common sense. Investing and planning for hard times in the future is sound counsel and advice. As King Solomon tells us in Proverbs 21:5 (ESV): "The plans of the diligent lead surely to abundance, but everyone who is hasty comes only to poverty."

By the time chemo was in full swing, my coworkers were deep in the Christmas season. I did not hear much from them, and I did not expect to hear either. From about early to mid-October, retail hours go up as shopping increases. Seasonal product sets change from back to school, to Halloween, to Thanksgiving/Christmas, to 100% Christmas within a few weeks. It is a nutty time in retail. It's hard to keep tabs on your own family during the holidays in retail. I was just a friend and coworker, so I did not expect any visits, phone calls, or cards.

After chemo ended, I did receive a phone call from the company, informing me that I no longer had a job with them. I had been replaced, and there was not anything that could be done. I recall wondering out loud how this information would look on the news; a cancer patient being fired for having cancer. It wasn't more than an hour later that I was told I had a job if I wanted one.

I am convinced that most employers try hard to be fair and honest with their employees, especially those who are on disability. I know companies have needs, stockholders have needs, and customers have needs that have to be met. I have run businesses, and know the pressures and exigencies of the corporate world. But frankly, everything is human to human, and ultimately spiritual. How a company treats employees is how it treats customers, stockholders, and each other. I would much rather work with companies that understand the Golden Rule, and operate by it, then anyone else.

During your cancer fight, is your employer supporting you?

If you are an employer, how can you better support employees who are suffering?

Do you know the Golden Rule? Do you believe it is still applicable today?

Matthew 7:12 (ESV), Jesus tells us, "So whatever you wish that others would do to you, do also to them, for this is the Law and the Prophets."

Chapter 21

I suppose a warning should be given at the beginning of this chapter. I have committed myself to be as accurate and transparent as possible about all aspects of my cancer, treatments, and my body's subsequent reaction to the treatments. This chapter focuses on a particularly gritty part of my treatment cycle. It is unpleasant, but true.

My first round of chemo went surprisingly well. Other than feeling bloated, I was able to keep exercising, and nausea was limited at first. I continued to walk a mile to a mile and a half every day, up and down and around the neighborhood. Thanksgiving came, and I was able to eat quite well, but not a ton as the bloating did affect my appetite. The turkey still tasted like turkey. The mashed potatoes tasted like whole milk and butter with a little potato thrown in. The cranberries were still tart and made my glands tingle.

At the beginning of my second cycle, my oncologist met with me. We went over my bloodwork, which was excellent. We covered my treatments and how I was handling them. She asked if I was exercising at all. I told her yes, I was still walking about a mile or so per day. My oncologist looked at me sharply and made a note. After the consultation, I was led over to my lounge chair. My nurses hooked me up to the IV and then went to get my chemo prescription for the day. I recall one of the nurses making a clucking noise with her tongue, and then she asked me to wait a moment as she wanted to confer with the oncologist. The nurse told me later that she was confirming the dosage increase—it was massive.

Apparently, being so physically active, while good for me, was an indication that I could take on more chemo. The more the better, I suppose, to make sure that any cancerous cells were killed off. I was given massive amounts of chemo in round two, and it completely kicked my butt. That week was cisplatin and etoposide, and then I was to come back on Monday and get the bleo. They also wanted to check my body and make sure I was handling the increase well.

The first week of my second greatly increased round of chemo ended up being brutal. My hair started to fall out by Friday. With the bleo, we knew the hair loss was likely to happen. Once the hair loss began, I carefully shaved my head. My plan all along was that if my hair started to fall out, I was going to take some control and choose to shave my head. When you have cancer, often there is not a lot of choice, so getting to choose when and how I went bald helped me cope mentally with the hair loss.

Besides the hair loss starting that week, my bloated feeling finally went away. On the Friday morning in question, I weighed 220 pounds at the oncologist's office. I felt as if I had a massive beer belly, or chemo belly, which I probably did. I drove home. I was still driving myself at the time, and I felt as if the seatbelt was pushing my stomach up into my throat. I felt miserable. This Friday night, when I arrived home, I noticed my hair falling into my sink, which is when I shaved my head. By the next morning, Saturday, all of the fluid that had built up in my body decided to come out. I had not thrown up until this point, but Saturday was a momentous day of projectile vomiting and diarrhea. I literally spent the next 24 hours in the bathroom evacuating what seemed to be all of my bodily fluids through two orifices. I barely peed; everything came out the other two routes.

I had never been that physically ill in my life. I admit I drank a lot in college, in what I call the Lost Years. But even then, after a weekend bender, I never came close to what those twenty-four hours were like with chemo. Once my body was totally drained, I looked like a scarecrow that the crows had picked clean. No beer belly, no nothing. I'm tempted to write that Sunday was a recovery day. It was a survival day. I just crashed. I barely moved. I did not eat, I did not drink. I just lay there immobile.

On Monday, somehow, and probably stupidly, I managed to drag myself downstairs to the car and drive myself to the oncology unit. Everyone at oncology noticed a massive change in me. I was not smiling; I was not joking. I shuffled when I walked, and I spoke in monosyllabic tones.

The nurses led me to my chemo chair so I could rest. After a little while, they helped me out of my chair and walked me over to the weigh-in center. They also took my blood pressure. I weighed 195 pounds. I recall looking at the number, thinking there was no way that was true. How could I have lost over 20 pounds in a weekend? My blood pressure was so low that the nurses went into ER mode. Three of them came over, held my arms and my waist, and then led me to the chair. As one of them said, "With that BP, you shouldn't be able to walk right now."

I settled into the chair, and quite frankly, I did not care about anything. I was so drained that there was not enough left of me to care about what was happening or what could happen. I just took it all in. My oncologist checked on me and then ordered a saline drip with potassium. I was told I would be in my chair all day. The saline plus potassium drip would take hours before it finished. If the potassium were administered too fast, it would kill me. In addition, I was given liquid potassium and other nutrients. My body was so dehydrated that I looked like, as one nurse later told me, the walking dead. They all debated whether I should be rushed to the local hospital or not. My oncologist conferred with me and we agreed I would be treated there, thank God.

I called my wife Laura to let her know I wouldn't be home by lunch. That was the original plan. I explained that I was in bad shape and would be in the chair for at least eight hours. Laura was not happy, and it was inconvenient. We had made a decision, months before, to go down to one vehicle. My work was within walking distance from our apartment. Her work was only a few miles away, so we figured it would save us a couple hundred a month in car payments, insurance, plates, and gas to have one car.

Laura was employed by a local artist who focused on AKC dog breeds. She was incredibly generous, gracious, and so nice about being flexible with our schedule that we were never concerned about Laura's job. As I recall, Laura's boss told her not to worry— she'd zoom in, pick her up, and take her home. At the time, Laura worked out of the artist's large home near Mt. Humphreys.

I spent the day in the chair, as predicted. I slept soundly for most of those eight hours. When I was done, I felt alive again. My eyeballs had felt gritty in their sockets that morning, as if I had sand in them. But after all of the fluid pumped back into me, my eyes felt normal again. The oncologist came and spoke with me for a while. If I had another attack like that again, the vomiting and diarrhea combo, I needed to call the nurse's line as soon as humanly possible. I had considered calling over the weekend but decided to wait until Monday.

For the rest of my treatments, I never did have another episode like that one again. Yes, I threw up again. In fact, I threw up a lot. Dear God, did I ever throw up. As she had read, Laura made two meals for me, one for me to eat and throw up, and another that I could keep down. Those second meals got smaller and smaller, and more simple, as the treatments wore on. At the outset of treatment, my oncologist and my nurses warned me that the chemo would cause extreme nausea and I would likely be vomiting quite a bit. Some people do not have nausea. I, however, did. With the chemo drugs I was taking, my body produced an over-abundance of the chemical serotonin, which caused my extreme nausea.

According to the National Cancer Institute, serotonin is "a hormone found in the brain, platelets, digestive tract, and pineal gland. It acts both as a neurotransmitter (a substance that nerves use to send messages to one another) and a vasoconstrictor (a substance that causes blood vessels to narrow)." Serotonin has been called "the happy chemical" because, in the right amount, it can cause a feeling of wellbeing. It is believed that too little serotonin can cause or contribute to depression. Too much serotonin, which is what happened for me, can cause nausea. My body was creating serotonin to push out the bad chemicals being pumped into my body. This excess serotonin affected the part of my brain that causes nausea, and in time it could cause depression as well. So with a lot of serotonin, I experience a lot of nausea.

The amount of times that I threw up was impressive. Each day, I did so at least three times. It became a routine, actually. I could sit at breakfast, be very hungry, wolf down a half a bowl of bland oatmeal, get up, say, "I'm going to throw up now," vomit for a few minutes, then come back, sit down, and eat toast with a little butter and maybe some natural jam, if I was up for it.

The weirdest thing, and this may be way too much to share, has to do with what happened when I had thrown up all the food in my stomach. I still am not quite sure what this was, but when my stomach was empty of all food, I was basically heaving up whatever chemical was left in my stomach. The color of the chemical or liquid was a bright orange, very similar to orange drink mix. I'm not suggesting it was serotonin, but every time that stuff came up, I thought, "I'm making so much serotonin, it's coming out of my mouth and nose." Chemo treatments and our reactions completely vary from person to person. I have known many people undergoing treatment who had almost no reactions or side effects. I did have side effects, and I had them in spades. When I think back on those times, and all of the awful reactions I had, there are two verses in Job that come to mind.

Did the author really need to be this transparent?

Does the reality and descriptions of real side effects of chemo help or hurt?

What is/was chemotherapy like for you?

Job 20:14–15 (ESV): "Yet his food is turned in his stomach; it is the venom of cobras within him. He swallows down riches and vomits them up again; God casts them out of his belly."

Chapter 22

Of the three drugs I was taking, the third drug, the one I took all on its own, was bleomycin. Bleo was given to me usually in week 2 or 3 of each cycle, if I remember correctly. The other two drugs, cisplatin and etoposide, were given at the same time, or at least during the same week.

Bleo is used in the treatments of various illnesses, including testicular, ovarian, Hodgkin's and non-Hodgkin's lymphoma, and other cancers and conditions. Bleo is considered to be an antitumor antibiotic. It is made from a type of fungus, and it attacks cancerous cells (and healthy ones) by stopping cell division. This is an incredibly simple description of a complicated process. Bleo helps keep cancers from growing and spreading, and thereby helps support other chemo drugs, to kill cancer (https://www.cancer.gov/about-cancer/treatment/drugs/bleomycin).

One of the major side effects of bleo is hair loss. It is also possible to have flu-like symptoms after having bleo administered. My first round went well, except for the hair loss. It was the second dose of bleo, during my second cycle, that did not go so well. After the extensive evacuation of all fluid from my body episode, my blood work showed that my immune system was incredibly weak. In particular, my white blood cell count was very low. With a weak immune system, I was susceptible to all manner of infections, and after the fluid evacuation episode, my medical team did not want to take any chances. So they decided that administering an immune booster would be appropriate.

After my second round of bleo treatment was finished, I was given a shot of a brand-name drug called Neupogen. This drug is designed to help my body produce more white blood cells. It is a good drug, and did help boost my immune system. What was not expected, however, was my reaction to Neupogen and to bleo. Bleo has a few side effects. As I have mentioned, hair loss is one. Nail thickening is another. Skin reactions are another potential side effect. The other one is fever and chills. On my first round of bleo, I had no side effects other than the hair loss. With this second dose, and with the Neupogen combined, I had a very strong reaction.

My understanding today is that oncologists do not administer bleo and Neupogen together. Instead, they wait at least 24 hours between administering both drugs. My experience was over fifteen years ago, so a lot has changed since then. In any event, my reaction to receiving both drugs on the same day came on very, very fast.

After the drugs were finished, and I was released from the oncology unit, I walked out to our car, started it up, and began driving home. About halfway up the mountain between Sedona and Flagstaff, just north of Oak Creek Canyon, I started to feel cold. It was late November or early December, so the temperature outside was around 40 degrees. Feeling cold was not unusual. I turned the car heater on to full. By the time I reached home, I was shivering uncontrollably and stumbled into bed.

Laura came home an hour later and found me curled up in bed, in a fetal position, shaking uncontrollably. My teeth were chattering so hard it was difficult to talk. Laura grabbed every blanket she could find and piled them on me. She also grabbed a space heater we kept for emergencies and put it on the floor, pointed right at my body. She turned it on full blast. I recall that our cat came in and lay on top of me, adding her warmth to the mix.

I do not remember exactly how long the chills lasted, but it was all evening and at least part of the night. I woke up the next morning feeling wrung out, like a rag that had been twisted until every drop of moisture had been squeezed out. It took me a few days to get over this reaction.

After this episode was over, Laura and I discussed what could have caused the chills and fever. With Neupogen being the only new addition to my regimen, we both assumed that it, coupled with bleo, had caused the side effects. We called the nurses' line and let them know about the side effects. They noted it and said chills were a potential side effect of the bleo, so we let it go. We should not have let this go, as I had two more rounds of bleo to go through.

How susceptible to side effects are you?

Do you know the contraindications of the drugs you take?

How well do you communicate these side effects to your physician?

1 Corinthians 3:16 (ESV): "Do you not know that you are God's temple and that God's Spirit dwells in you?"

Chapter 23

Once I was diagnosed with cancer, Laura conducted a ton of research. The day after I was diagnosed, we went to the Flagstaff Public Library, which is one of the best libraries I have ever spent time in. Laura and I grew up in small to mid-sized towns in Indiana, and the public library system was fundamental to our education. My small school had one of my favorite librarians, and she used to feed me books. Whenever she got a new shipment in, Fran would select out one or two books for me as well as for a few other kids. Her selections were always dead on. When we moved to Flagstaff, we became members of the public library as soon as we could. Their selection of titles was impressive, and it fit our needs and wants as if we had selected the books ourselves. The day after the diagnosis, we spent hours in the library, each following our own strategy.

I selected several technical books on cancer, as well as two books written by people who either had testicular cancer or who had been touched by it. Laura took the nutritional approach. She pored over books about diet and nutritional supplements. When we left, we had about ten books between us. It was this research, along with the information our doctors had given us, that allowed Laura to put her battle plan together.

I call it a battle plan because that is exactly what it was. Laura set a goal—total healing—which included my ability to naturally father children once the chemo was finished. She built a diet plan of foods that would give me maximum nutritional value while limiting any kind of dietary substance that might help the cancer grow. In addition to meal plans, she listed out and found natural vitamins, minerals, and fungi that other cultures (in particular Japan) used as natural remedies or system boosters during chemo.

We, of course, ran the meal plans and the supplements past our oncologist. She was impressed with and approved of Laura's battle plan. My diet change was immediate and enduring. No more processed sugars, no more processed foods, no dairy desserts—just whole food, as natural as could be. Luckily, Flagstaff has a great farmer's market, so we were able to eat whole foods. We kept to chicken and turkey rather than beef or pork, absolutely no hot dogs, and we decided to stay away from fish, just to be safe. There were mercury content warnings for fish at the time.

Whenever we cooked a chicken or turkey, we rubbed the skin down with a little olive oil and not much else. Once chemo started and the vomiting kicked in, I did not eat a lot of food, but what I did eat was nutrient rich. I kept up with the supplements until the final cycle. That's when I hit rock bottom.

The medical staff we worked with was very supportive of our battle plan. However, we did run into people every now and then who did not believe in what we were doing. I had a scan set up for late December, and when we went in to get registered, the admin and the tech asked me about certain supplements I was taking. In particular, the tech very politely asked me why I was taking folic acid. Pregnant women do, but why would I? Laura had read that folic acid could have a positive effect on my sperm count. I told the tech we wanted to have more children when the chemo was over, and folic acid was one of the supplements we believed would help us do so naturally.

The lady actually laughed at the prospect of us having more children naturally. She recovered quickly, but she was not the only person to challenge our thinking. Others would look at us as if we were grasping at straws. Laura and I believed in what we were doing, and we approached it faithfully. We prayed about it, did the research, and followed a path we believed would help us get through chemo and help me to be as healthy as possible post-chemo.

We prayed about the battle plan as much as we did everything else. We kept in mind Paul's admonition in Philippians 4:6: "Do not be anxious about anything, but in everything by prayer and supplication with thanksgiving let your requests be made known to God." We let our requests be known to Him, that is for certain.

Near the end of chemo, there were a few circumstances that made following the battle plan challenging. The nausea, as I mentioned earlier, had gotten so severe that even the second meal was getting harder and harder to keep down, and the cisplatin had a strange effect on my taste buds. Everything I ate tasted coppery or metallic—not a vague taste either, but a strong one, similar to sucking on a brand-new penny.

When the nausea and the metal taste got so bad, there were two things we turned to that helped see me through the final weeks of chemo. The first were natural lemon Chiclets; they were a godsend. Someone suggested them, and the sharp lemon flavor overpowered the metallic taste. The Chiclets were sugar free, and the flavor did not overstay its welcome like other candy. The second item that helped sustain me when I could not get anything else to stay down in my stomach was a generic chocolate-flavored milk drink that was packed with vitamins, minerals, and calories. This chocolate drink was not in the original battle plan as the sugar content was high. However, near the end of my chemo cycle, we tried a bunch of different food products (yogurt, toast, juices, etc.) that I could not keep down. The only one I could keep down that had nutrients, and was sweet enough to cut through the metallic taste, was the chocolate drink. I must have drunk gallons of the stuff. Yes, I was still throwing up, but the drink had the added benefit of being easy on me when it came up, and for whatever reason, I did not have an issue drinking another glass, after I threw up the first.

I am not suggesting the chocolate drink was a great solution, nor am I recommending it to anyone else. I am not a doctor, after all. I am only mentioning the drink as when the nausea was at its highest, and nothing could stay down, we did not give up on finding an answer. Never give up, keep fighting, keep looking; there is something out there that can help sustain you physically.

Physically, a children's chocolate drink sustained me. Spiritually, God continued to sustain me.

Have you ever had to radically change your diet? What happened?

What is the most important life event you have planned for? How did it go?

What are your short- and long-term health goals? How are you going to achieve them?

Psalm 63:1 (ESV): "O God, you are my God; earnestly I seek you; my soul thirsts for you; my flesh faints for you, as in a dry and weary land where there is no water."

Chapter 24

Have you ever been prompted to pray for someone with no known reason as to why? Have you ever been awakened at night, unable to go back to sleep, thinking of someone in particular for some unknown reason? Maybe someone you have not seen or even thought of for years? Have you ever prayed for days, weeks, or months for someone, with no discernible results? You may even believe those prayers are falling on deaf ears or are ineffective. Have you ever wondered about the effectiveness of prayer?

After the episode of nonstop chills, and after the seemingly total evacuation of the fluids from my body, I hit a very hard mental wall, and not for the last time. In hindsight, there were times when I realized I was in despair. Despair can be defined as a complete absence of hope, and that is what I felt. Even after the amazing gift God gave me by revealing Himself to me (at least partially), the blackness, the void of hope, hit me. There was a night at the end of my second cycle of chemo, probably during week five, where true despair hit.

During my treatments, I became quite accomplished, I thought, at concealing how I really felt. My oncology nurses always asked me how I was feeling, and I was nearly always able to answer brightly with an "I'm OK." Laura knew me better, and she never accepted this response as true. I suppose the nurses knew as well.

On this particular day, I had been in a dark mood—not angry, just dark. I was brooding, and could not get my mind out of it. Laura got on me that day about being honest with my nurses about how I was feeling, not just physically, but also mentally. She was concerned about my mental well being. We were reaching the halfway point of my treatments, and she was fighting to keep me focused and sane.

My son, who had the uncanny ability to brighten up any room on any day, was failing to brighten me up. I was so down that I did not want to pray. I did not want to read the Bible. I did not want to think. I just wanted it, all of it, to be over. Despair is a hard feeling to describe. The closest I can get is a poor analogy.

Imagine being in a room with four hallways, arrayed on each point of the compass. The room is dimly lit, just enough to see that there are hallways leading out and that they are all dark and foreboding. The room itself is dangerous to be in, and any step could be fatal. You want out of the room, but you cannot see a clear pathway, even when you know the paths are there. Everything you need to get out of the room is there for you, but you cannot see it. Everywhere you look is darkness, and the light you have is just enough to juxtapose the darkness. The darkness is emphasized and is overpowering the light. The point is that a part of me knew that the answer out of the despair was at hand; I just could not see it. I went to bed this night and there was nothing but darkness in my mind. I lay down next to my wife, unsure of what would be next, unsure of another day. I had not prayed all day; in fact, it had been a few days since I had done so. As I lay there with this darkness swirling around and through me, a scripture broke through the darkness. The scripture was an image from Sunday school of Peter walking out to Jesus on the water in Matthew 14:30: "But when he [Peter] saw the wind, he was afraid, and beginning to sink, he cried out, 'Lord, save me.'"

All I could pray at that moment was "Lord, save me." Anything more would have been too difficult. When I prayed, "Lord, save me," at that very moment, the despair left me, and I felt I was back in the light again. Not only did the despair lift like a veil, but another image also entered my mind.

As I prayed that simple prayer, which was answered immediately, a picture of my Little League coach's wife, Sandy, entered my mind. The image popping in was the weirdest thing. I had not thought of Joe or Sandy for years, even though we all considered each other family. We played baseball together growing up, went to church camp together, and attended the same church for a while. In fact, my parents attended the same church as Joe and Sandy did at the time. It was inexplicable.

A few days later, I was still back in the light. Mom and I had a call. While I was going through the cancer fight, I had regularly scheduled calls with my family back in Indiana. My brother was every Sunday afternoon. My grandfather was every Thursday. My parents were on Fridays or Saturdays, sometimes on a Monday.

During this call with my mom, I shared with her the despair from a few nights before, my prayer, and how it left me so suddenly. Almost in passing, I mentioned that I had a picture of Sandy pop in my head at that time. I told her I could not figure out why I had thought of Sandy at that moment.

Mom got really quiet and stayed quiet. I asked, "Mom?" thinking we had been cut off.

Mom said, "I think I know why."

On Sunday, Sandy had approached Mom during the "meet & greet" part of the service. Mom and Dad's church was medium sized, so at the beginning of the service, after the first hymn was sung, everyone would mill around shaking hands, hugging people, welcoming visitors, and checking in with each other. During that Sunday's service, Sandy had sought Mom out. She told my mom that God had awakened her early one morning and laid it on her heart to pray for me. Sandy told Mom when she woke up, God made it plain to her that she was to get up out of bed, kneel at the bed, and pray for me, as if I were her own son. And being the God-loving Christian she is, Sandy did it. She obeyed, and she shared with my mom that she prayed for an hour at her bedside.

Mom and I talked about what night this was and about what time. The day and the time matched up. Sandy was praying for me during one of my darkest hours. Sandy lived 1,700 miles away from me. We had not spoken in years. Yet God chose her, and probably others, to pray for me. And her obedience to God, His will, and His calling helped deliver me from the despair. James tells us: "The prayer of a righteous person has great power, as it is working" (James 5:16b). The idea is that the person praying has an intense and sincere confidence in God, or simply put, prays in great faith. When a righteous person prays, someone who believes and has accepted Christ Jesus as their Lord and Savior, that prayer has great power.

Months later, when I visited home and attended their church, I sought Sandy out and shared what happened to me and how I felt the despair lift as someone prayed for me. She exclaimed, "It was me!" and we both cried and rejoiced that God had used her to help me in my time of need.

My friend, if you are praying for someone, do not stop. Keep praying, and keep praying expectantly. Trust in Him and be confident that He will answer you. The days may be long, and His answer may not be what you expect, but He will answer. And if you are awakened in the middle of the night and you cannot sleep, ask God who you should be praying for, and then do it. That person needs your prayers. You may never ever know what effect your prayer may have had on this earth, but trust me, your prayers are not wasted.

Have you ever despaired? What was it like for you?

Have you ever been compelled to pray for someone?

Who can you pray for today? Who came to mind as you read this chapter?

Job 24:22 (ESV): "Yet God prolongs the life of the mighty by his power; they rise up when they despair of life."

Chapter 25

I wish I could say my mental state was stable throughout the remainder of my chemo treatments. I wish I could say it, but I cannot, as it would be untrue. On a Sunday night, the Sunday before I started my third round of chemo, I could feel the despair creeping in again. I prayed and went to bed thinking it would be OK. I was halfway through, and I needed to think about the remaining treatments this way. Instead, I began brooding again.

By morning, and after Laura and my son had left, I was dragging physically and mentally. It was a struggle to get out of bed and go out the door, let alone get down the stairs. When I reached the car, I just sat in the driver's seat for several minutes. I remember looking at the clock thinking I needed to get going; otherwise, I would be late. So I started the car and headed down the road. By the time I left the parking lot, I was in a very dark place. The next two cycles of chemo were daunting. I felt so bad now, how could I get through six more weeks? The road I drove down to my treatments was 89A. It is a long, winding road. It starts out at around 7,000 feet and drops down to 5,000. The road takes many twists and turns as it goes down the mountain into Oak Creek Canyon. There is a lot of natural beauty, and there are many natural dropoffs along this road.

The thought entered my mind at the first major switchback down to Sedona. What if the car drove over the edge? The drop was enough to end it all. The thought was nothing more than that, a thought, but the casualness of the thought terrified me. Then the thought came again with the unhelpful addition: it would be quick. The addition was disturbing. I tried pushing these thoughts away and focused on driving, but they kept coming back.

By the time I had driven through the switchbacks, I was getting comfortable with the idea of taking my own life. With each thought, the fear, the terror, and the wrongness of it lessened and lessened. By the time I saw the first bridge abutment, I nearly had myself convinced. At the next bridge, the thought came I should unhook the seat belt, accelerate, turn the wheel a bit, and be done with this mess.

When the second abutment came, I reached for my seatbelt and pressed the accelerator. As soon as the engine revved, a cold fear instantly grabbed me. I took my foot off the accelerator and put both shaking hands back on the wheel. *Dear God,* I prayed. *Help me!* I cried. I prayed out loud and began to tell God He had to do something. I could not handle this. It was too much. He had to do it. And I asked Him to forgive me for what I had almost done. I prayed in anger at myself and at God that I would reach this state. I was as angry at Him as I could be.

I prayed until I drove into the parking lot of the oncology unit. I was early, so I prayed in the car, still angry but oh, so tired. I dragged myself out of the car and trudged in. *Six more weeks,* I kept thinking. *Six more weeks.* When I entered the unit, the smell hit me immediately.

Oncology units the world over have a heavy chemical odor to them. It smells to me like a cross between saline, copper, and weed killer. When I caught the scent upon entering the door, I walked immediately to the men's room and threw up. I'll spare the detail here, but just know this was the first time I threw up at the unit. After this day, every subsequent trip to the unit during my treatments, I threw up every time I smelled the chemicals.

After throwing up and cleaning myself up, I checked in. A nurse was waiting for me. She was bright and cheerful. She commented how good the color in my cheeks was.

My response: "I just threw up."

"Oh," she said.

Instead of leading me to the chair, she led me back to one of the examining rooms. She asked me the normal questions, to which I answered, "OK" to each one. I did this a lot. People would ask sincerely, "How are you?" The honest answer that day was I'd just considered killing myself with my car, but instead I said, "OK." This was and is a mistake. It is OK to not be OK and to admit it.

It is OK to be honest with yourself and with your medical staff to say, "I'm not OK." Cancer is messy and horrible. Shoot, life is messy, and sometimes we are not OK. I'm a fixer; I like to fix things, but I could not fix this. I should have been more honest.

After the nurse left, my oncologist came in. She asked me all the same questions, and I gave the same answers. She clearly did not believe me. After the questions, she gave me a physical. When she was finished, she had me get off the examination table and asked me to sit in a chair. Then she went over my bloodwork. Her back was to me, and I was waiting for her to challenge me on how I was really feeling.

Instead of challenging me, she wrote down several notes and then casually said, "You are doing extremely well." She paused and then turned to look me in the eye, surprising me by saying, "You are doing so well, in fact, that this week plus your bleo will be your last round."

Her words hit me hard emotionally. I cried. I sat in the chair and cried. My oncologist just reached over and put her hand on my knee and waited until I could talk. I asked her to repeat what she had said. I wanted to make sure I had heard her correctly. She confirmed that I was now on my last round of chemo. I cried some more and then I stood up, and she hugged me. When I walked in,

I was dead inside. After this surprise, after God answered again, I skipped to my chemo chair.

God's timing is nearly never on our schedule. We have to trust Him regardless. As followers of Jesus, we have to trust Him when we cannot see His hand or divine His purpose, or when He does not meet our expectations. God has shown up for me so often and so explicitly that I must be a slow learner or something. At my worst moment, and the drive in was the worst moment of my cancer, He seemingly was not there, but He was. He was not just with me; He was also ahead of me, like always.

When I called Laura after the treatment, I was ebullient. I had a joy that alarmed her.

When she heard me on the call, she immediately asked, "What's wrong?" It took some time for me to get my emotions under control, but I eventually got it out. She could not believe it. She knew how bad I had been, and her prayers were sustaining me more than I can probably ever know. We both rejoiced and I was able to play with my son for the first time in weeks. I still felt horrible physically, but mentally and spiritually I was totally new.

Have you struggled with depression or suicidal thoughts?

Is there someone you can talk to—a friend, a colleague, a counselor?

Promise you won't act without talking to this person, even if it is an internal promise. Do not act on any self destructive thoughts. Be sure to talk to someone. People love you and want to help you; please let them!

2 Peter 3:9 (ESV): "The Lord is not slow to fulfill His promise as some count slowness but is patient toward you, not wishing that any should perish, but that all should reach repentance."

Chapter 26

The last cycle of chemo went well. We were approaching Christmas by this time, and my treatments would be completed shortly afterward. We had plans for a trip to Seattle post-chemo, leaving sometime in mid-January. Laura and I with our son, all of us, needed to get away. My sister-in-law and her husband live in Seattle. It is our favorite place to visit outside of northern Arizona. It has great food and great music. It is a beautiful city with lots to see and do.

With Christmas approaching, and my chemo winding down, Laura started to plan for dinner on Christmas Eve. Back then, we always had duck, either on Christmas Eve or Christmas Day. We were going over to our friends' house to celebrate on Christmas Day, so our dinner plans were for Christmas Eve.

I had an appointment with the oncologist Christmas Eve morning. I did not think much of it. I thought the appointment was to be simple bloodwork, followed by bleo, then home. When I arrived, I felt well, especially considering the previous nine weeks. I did my normal routine: entered through the front door, went to the men's room, and threw up—fortunately, this time it was light. Then I went to check in, got my blood draw completed, and waited in the chair for the bleo. There was no Benadryl given this time, just the bleo. When the bleo drip was through, after maybe fifteen minutes, one of the oncology nurses came over with a shot. I asked her what the shot was for, and she answered, "It's Nuepogen; your WBC count is low again." Then she gave me the shot.

I immediately thought about the reaction last time. What could I do? I could not tell her to not give me the shot. I should have asked to speak to the doctor about the reaction, but it was too late. Once the shot was administered, I was wished a Merry Christmas, and then I checked out. By the time I got to the car, I was already shaking.

I started the car, turned the heat on full, and put on a coat that was in the backseat. The chills were setting in quickly, and they were so bad that I was not sure I would be able to make it home safely. I prayed and prayed. I thought about calling Laura, but I knew how upset this was going to make her. Christmas dinner was in my mind when I remembered how the last time I had this reaction, it took a full day to recover.

My prayers were for her, and to get the chills over with as early as possible, so we could not only make it to our friends' house on Christmas Day, but so we could also have dinner that night. I made it home safely. The trip seemed to take forever as I had to focus hard on every mile of the drive. It was an ugly trip, with me shaking the whole way.

As soon as I got home, I went to bed, piling on the blankets, and putting the space heater right next to my side of the bed. I prayed I would go to sleep and wake up better. I did not want this last gasp of my treatments to disappoint Laura at her favorite time of the year. Laura grew up in a big family, and Christmas was a family-rich tradition for her. Since we had been together, we had created many traditions of our own. Today, Christmas Eve is the night we open our first presents, always new pajamas. We eat subs and chips and watch a Christmas movie or special. On Christmas Day, we have a menu that's been set for decades now. Back in 2002, the main course was duck; today it's prime rib. We have a lot of people come over for Christmas dinner now, and a duck or two just is not quite enough to go around.

After weeks and months of surgeries and chemotherapy, we had turned the corner finally, and Christmas was to be a big celebration of the end of chemotherapy. Instead, I was having another reaction, lying in bed covered in blankets, the space heater going full blast, and our cat curled up by my head, all while I was shaking uncontrollably. I cannot imagine how Laura felt, the disappointment or the sadness at our celebration being delayed a few days. Laura had been so strong and such a stalwart during this entire fight. I hated that I was laid up again.

I was half asleep when Laura came home. She walked into the bedroom and asked me what was wrong. I told her they gave me Neupogen with my bleo today. I think she ranted a bit, and then I told her I was going to sleep and try to get better.

When I was on chemo, I did not dream very much. I had a few dreams, but nothing I recall. I do remember a dream this Christmas Eve. In the dream, I was in bed, in our apartment, and I saw a shaft of golden light come crashing down and literally explode in the living room. It was so bright that I could see the brightness through the walls, spilling through all of the doorways of the apartment. It seemed so real and was so bright that this image woke me from a deep sleep. I sat up in bed, curious, as the light reminded me of the light from the bathroom, back at the beginning of this entire affair. I got up out of bed and realized I felt better. In fact, I felt awesome. I was tired, a little sore, but I was also hungry, and I wanted to eat some duck.

Walking out of the bedroom, I found Laura lying on the couch. I must have surprised her as she jumped up. "What?" she asked, expecting something awful.

I remember smiling as I told her I was hungry. I walked into the kitchen, looking for the duck. Laura followed me in, and the look on her face was of total incredulity. She had thrown the small duck into the oven and cooked it, but she had not done much else. She expected me to be down and out for the night, so she had not put much together. I pulled it out of the oven, and we finished the duck together. I felt bloated but happy.

A few years later, we were sitting around the table with our pastor and his wife (Pastor Doug and Kathy at the time) from our new church. I was telling them about my experiences and all of the amazing things God did for us, and when I was through, Laura started to speak. She had never mentioned this to me before, but that night, Christmas Eve night, when I was sick again, all of the previous few months, the weight of them, came crashing down on her—the emotion, the fear, the disappointment, all of it, all at once. She shared with us that on that Christmas Eve night, it was all too much for her. Our dinner plans were ruined. Her favorite time of the year was spoiled. The disappointment of it all became too much. Laura gave it all over to God, admitting she could not handle it herself, and put her full faith and trust in Him.

I tell people I am thankful that I went through cancer. And I am thankful, for a lot of reasons. The primary reason, though, is that cancer brought me closer to Him, and more importantly, my wife, Laura, came to a saving knowledge of Him.

What leads you or is leading you to fully trust Christ?

Do you trust Him in everything?

Have you trusted Him for your salvation?

The Apostle Paul tells us in **Romans 10:9-10** (ESV): "If you declare with your mouth, 'Jesus is Lord,' and believe in your heart that God raised him from the dead, you will be saved. For it is with your heart that you believe and are justified, and it is with your mouth that you profess your faith and are saved."

Chapter 27

Around the end of my chemotherapy treatments, several events occurred that led us to consider moving back to Indiana. We had lived in Arizona for over three years and loved it there. We still do, but we came to believe we were being led back to Indiana.

On my original CT scan and subsequent i131 uptake tests, a cold nodule was confirmed to be on my thyroid. The i131 test consists of radioactive iodine being ingested. The thyroid uses iodine, in part, to manufacture the hormones it produces. By taking the radioactive iodine, and then scanning the thyroid a day or so later, doctors can determine how much iodine the thyroid used, which helps them spot cold nodules and other potential issues in the thyroid. The test confirmed that a cold nodule could be serious, or it could be nothing. Once my chemo was nearing an end, my oncologist had my original surgeon set up a needle biopsy on the cold nodule.

A needle biopsy is when a medical professional takes a syringe with a very long needle, sticks it into your body and then into a mass, removes some tissue with the syringe, and then has the tissue analyzed. In this case, the long needle went into my neck from the side. It was relatively painless. I just had to stay completely still.

The biopsy itself went well. The test results did not. About a week after the needle biopsy, the surgeon's office called me and asked me to come in. The tone of the call was somber, which told me the news would not be good. Laura and I went in that day, a few hours after the call. We sat and waited for my surgeon and nurse practitioner to come in. I was not exactly nervous, just waiting for whatever was to come.

When my surgeon came in, he was able to convey with a single look that he had bad news. The look on my nurse practitioner's face was one of great concern and worry. After saying hello, they got right to the point. My biopsy had revealed that I had the early stages of papillary thyroid cancer.

Papillary thyroid cancer, according to the National Cancer Institute, is the most common thyroid cancer. It has a high survival rate; 90% of diagnosed individuals live more than ten years. It is curable and has a stated protocol. I was to be given some time to recover from chemotherapy and enjoy our vacation to Seattle, and then as soon as I got back, I would have part of my thyroid removed, and radiation treatments would be administered thereafter.

Right before my thyroid cancer diagnosis, I was trying to figure out if I was going to go back to work or not. January 31, 2003, was supposed to be the end of disability for me, which meant I needed to go back to work. I was not ready for it, and honestly, I did not want to work in retail anymore. After all of the treatments, the idea of working 60+ hours a week did not interest me at all. I was praying diligently about God providing a solution. I believe in His way, He did.

After the thyroid diagnosis, I was none too pleased with His solution. I took the news calmly and stayed calm for a few hours. Then, when we got home, I lost it. I went on a very long, very curse-laden tirade about God and His plans. I was angry and afraid. I had not seen this second cancer coming—who would?—and I just went off. Laura listened for a bit and then left the room. I didn't blame her.

When I was done with this tirade, I remembered my prayer about not going back to work, and it ticked me off. How in the world was I going to go back to work and fight this cancer, too? What kind of answer was this?

I went and saw my general practitioner for a checkup the next day. I mentioned work to him, and he looked at me as if I were a complete idiot. He then proceeded to lecture me about thinking I was some kind of superhuman or a professional athlete. He wondered if I had learned anything about being with family, and then he extended my disability through June 30th. I was to get my thyroid cancer treated and then take a few months off.

After all of the challenges and this latest blow, and also being well aware of the challenging job market in Flagstaff, I would be coming off cancer and competing against MBAs for the right level of positions. It was at this point in mid-January that I started thinking about making a move. I explored jobs in Seattle, Wyoming, Idaho, and back in Indiana. Regardless, I felt doors were closing in Arizona. The older couple who had adopted us in Flagstaff agreed; they believed doors were closing as well.

On a lark, I checked out rental trucks. This was January, so prices were actually pretty cheap. I was able to reserve a truck for June 30, 2003, which would be my last day at my current employer and on our apartment rental agreement. Laura and I discussed a potential move, and while we prepared for the possibility, we were not altogether in agreement. So, like everything else, we prayed about it for a long time.

The thyroid surgery went well. The surgeon took one look at my thyroid and removed the whole thing. He did not want to take any chances. It was a tricky procedure, as my laryngeal nerve was located in an unusual spot. I could have lost my voice entirely or come out sounding all gravelly-toned. Laura was not opposed to me possessing a more gravelly voice.

The surgery was scheduled to be relatively short, so I was a bit surprised when I awoke in my room and saw that several hours had passed. Why I would be surprised by anything, I do not know. My surgeon and nurse practitioner were waiting for me to wake up. Usually I had to wait for them to come in after I woke up. Instead, they were already there. They both said hello. I said hello back, and I could see both of them visibly relax and audibly breathe a sigh of relief. The location of my laryngeal nerve made the surgeon take his time, and he was a bit concerned.

My anesthesiologist for the surgery was one of my good friends from church. I am thankful for him being in the operating room with me. I had a follower of Christ in there with me, praying throughout. He told me later he had never seen a surgeon take so much care before; they are usually in and out, effective and efficient, but my surgeon did not hurry this time. He opened me up, took one look, and then methodically and slowly did the work. I am thankful for all of the medical staff, of course, but it amazed me that God put one of His people in my corner, praying right by the surgeon.

The radiation therapy was a few weeks later, post-surgery. Again, they took no chances; I was given a large dose of radioactive iodine that would be taken up by any surviving thyroid cells and would subsequently destroy them. Other doctors have looked at the dosage they gave me of radioactive iodine, and all of them confirmed that it was an impressively large dose. I did not glow in the dark, but I did get to stay in an isolation room for 48 hours. Everything I brought in with me to that room had to be burned afterward. So I brought two books, read them, and then allowed them to be burned.

In hindsight, the time I was able to spend alone reading two of C.S. Lewis's best books was necessary and helped clear my mind. When I came out of isolation, both Laura and I knew it was time to move on.

What is the biggest decision you have ever had to make?

How did your faith inform your decision?

How did you ask Him for guidance?

1 John 5:14 (ESV): "And this is the confidence that we have toward Him, that if we ask anything according to His will He hears us."

Chapter 28

Once our decision was made to move back to Indiana, we began making a lot of calls and had further discussions. Laura and I debated what part of Indiana we would settle in. I was comfortable moving back to northern Indiana, where we grew up; or even southern Indiana, where we went to college. Laura wanted to move to Indianapolis. After researching jobs and housing, and after a lot of prayer, we decided on Indianapolis. The job market was large and we were more likely to find work quickly.

We also decided we were finished living in apartments, so we started looking at rental houses online. We also had friends who lived in Indy look at houses for us. Eventually, a month or two before the move, we were able to find a house, get the money sent over for a deposit, and put the housing need to bed.

With a truck and a house settled, my doctors and I discussed the move back. They all understood that our family was back in Indiana. With no real job prospects in Flagstaff, we were making a good decision for our little family. Our son had no idea what was going on. He only knew we were moving and that he would be closer to his grandparents. He was not even two years old yet. He was very excited that his paternal grandfather was coming out to visit us before the move.

Laura and I thought through and planned the move to Indiana. Since all of us could not fit in the truck, and we did not want to drive our car back, which would enable us to save on additional gas money, we decided the best scenario was to have Laura fly back with our son a few days early, sign the final house rental papers, and get the key to the house. This way, when my dad and I arrived with the truck, everyone would be ready to go and we could start unloading right away. We had assembled a large number of people to help us unload the truck when we arrived in Indiana. The plan of Laura being on hand early to coordinate would be very, very helpful.

I asked Dad to drive cross-country with me because, while I did feel healthy, I was not sure how fit I would be to drive a large truck, with a car towed behind it, for over 1,600 miles, especially since part of it was in the mountains. Dad had owned his own trucking company for a few decades, so he was very experienced and ready to help. He was eager in fact, since he hated us living so far away.

My grandfather was delighted when I told him we were moving back. He kept asking us about money and whether we would be OK financially or not. I had not worked in over nine months, and money had to be a problem, he was thinking. Well, money was a problem. We were running out of cash, and when the disability ran out, we would be out of any kind of income. We were moving across the country without jobs. And we had just signed a lease, which meant we needed to start making $900 a month in payments. Our level of financial difficulty was pretty darn high, but again, we were trusting in God and being obedient to Him.

The drive across the country went off without a hitch. The only hiccup we had was with our cat. She kept overheating in the truck. She was in a cat carrier in the cab, but she could not receive a good airflow, so we kept the windows open most of the time. We stayed at two hotels on the drive back, and she kept mewling all night, but we all survived.

Laura and our son, however, missed their flight. Laura's artist employer had miscalculated the drive down from Flagstaff to Phoenix International Airport, among other things. My wife and son ended up missing a direct flight to Indy, and they had to wait for a later flight. The later flight was not direct, so they ended up making several unexpected stops between Phoenix and Indy. I heard later on how exhausted they both were. They got back to Indiana before we did, but just barely.

The day we arrived in Indiana was wonderful. I remember crossing the border from Illinois and feeling contentment. We were finally home. I loved Arizona and still do. We go back to Flagstaff as often as we can, but Indiana is home. We arrived right before the Fourth of July weekend, so as soon as we had unloaded the truck, returned it to the rental agency, and locked up our little house, we headed back up north to spend the weekend with our families.

On this visit, my grandfather had asked me and my mom if I could go on a "spree" with him when we were back home. A spree with grandpa meant I'd be in his truck and we could end up anywhere. When I was little, I would go with him on these sprees quite often. We would go as far south as Indianapolis, as far west as Rochester, and as far north as Nappanee or Shipshewana. We had a great time whenever we were together. Most of these trips were spent with Grandpa sharing stories from when he was a kid and talking about scripture, IU basketball, or about how to make and save money every day.

This particular spree after our return home was very special and is a cherished memory of mine. I thought he was going to have me load dog food (he used to sell it as a side business). Instead, we drove around in the country. And we just talked. Grandpa had missed me terribly and I him. It was just the two of us chatting and driving. We stopped and had coffee at a little diner we both knew. The diner hadn't changed much in the years we had lived in Arizona. Grandpa and I enjoyed the time we got to spend together. We were home.

After this first weekend together with the whole family, we drove back to Indy and settled into a routine. I began to job hunt, and Laura did the same. I also had a yard to maintain for the first time in years, so at first, I would mow and detail the yard. Each day I would take our son for a long walk, miles in fact. We had a backpack he could ride in. We would start out together, walk as far as I could, and then turn back. I was working on getting back into good physical shape.

My son and I loved our time together. I also started writing résumés and filling out job applications by the score. While there were a lot of jobs available in Indianapolis, it turned out that we needed to know people to get an interview. I probably applied for over 500 jobs from July to October that year. And I settled into a depression with each passing failed job application. I kept praying and trusting, but the number of rejections piled up fast. I should have known God was going before me again.

Have you ever suffered job loss?

What was it like for you?

Is your identity in your job or in Christ?

Deuteronomy 31:8 (ESV): "It is the Lord who goes before you. He will be with you; he will not leave you or forsake you. Do not fear or be dismayed."

Chapter 29

The first summer back in Indiana was a long one. Each day seemed to roll into the next, excruciatingly slowly. Each day meant no calls for interviews and no responses to job applications. Each passing day meant finding and making job applications, résumé submissions, phone calls, and emails, all of which were fruitless. Each day meant rejections. Laura and I began to fight a lot. She was not so much upset about the lack of a job and a lack of an income as much as my mood and mental state. I was taking these rejections personally (which is a mistake, as it is almost never personal).

I hate money. I really do. And it was at this time in my life that I learned to despise its necessity. Each day without a job meant a day without income. We did have medical bills. We had our rent to pay and other bills, such as utilities. The weight of the bills and lack of income was ever present. At the time, I still had my identity, how I saw myself, which was centered on how much money I could make or in the job that I held. I was wrong in my thinking.

My identity should be, and is, in Christ. He lived, died, and rose, all so that I and anyone else who calls upon Him can be with Him. There is no greater identity than this: I am a child of God. I am His. Jesus died for me and for all of us, so we may have an identity in Him, if we so choose.

During this time, God was so incredibly generous with us. Each day I would get mail from off the porch and find rejection letters, bills, or even worse, no responses to the myriad applications I submitted. But every now and then, I would go to the mailbox on our porch and I would find a letter with something unexpected inside: money.

One letter came from the medical offices back in Flagstaff, informing us that Laura and I had overpaid: "Here's a $600 refund." Or I would get a letter from my former employer's pension fund: "Since your fund was under $10,000, here is a check for $7,000." Or I would receive a check for unused vacation time or for whatever. We literally had money pour in, always when we needed it most, and always from sources we never expected. It was crazy how God provided for us. In the Old Testament, one of the many names the nation of Israel called God was Jehovah Jireh. The name means "The Lord Will Provide." In His providence, He was not just providing for us financially. He has done this for many of His saints. He was also providing for our daily needs physically and spiritually.

There is an autobiography by George Müller that is incredibly inspiring and challenges me every time I hear or read about him and his life. George Müller was a missionary in England back in the early part of the 1800s. He worked with orphans, and his stories of God's daily provision are amazing.

For his mission work, George Müller resolved to not ask people for money or donations. Instead, he relied upon God for all of his, his wife's, and the orphans' needs. One of the stories he shares in his autobiography tells about the day they ran out of milk, and the orphans would not have any for their breakfast of oatmeal. George Müller, his wife, and some employees began to pray, asking God for their need, and while they were yet praying (see Daniel 9), a knock came at the door. It was a letter with money, enough to buy milk, and then other letters arrived, all with money or pledges of funds to sustain the orphanage. All of these came unbidden, save for the request they put fully to God.

God does provide. We often equate God's provision with money, and yes, I have benefited greatly at my hour of need from God's provision, but He offers us so much more. He offers us an eternity with Him, if we just choose Him. I often think God provides for us in this way, monetarily, because we find it easy to measure. I am grateful every time, but wish money were not such a necessity here.

My job search went on until mid-October. As so often happens with me, I was focused on my doing this instead of allowing God to lead. The day came where I just let go of any idea of trying to control this situation. I walked into my office (the small third bedroom in our rental) and sat down. Instead of looking for a job online or in the paper, I prayed. I prayed, and God led me. After praying I looked down, and on the floor was an open phone book directory.

For those who do not know what a phone directory was, back in 2003, while cell phones were in rampant use then, they were not exactly smart. The first smartphone hit the market in 1992, but they were not ubiquitous until after June 2007. Without an internet connection at our fingertips, we had to rely upon physical phone directories that listed our home phone number. The directories also provided businesses with an avenue to advertise, in a section called the Yellow Pages.

When I looked down, the phone book was open to the Yellow Pages, specifically the employment section. The page displayed was a half-page ad for a temp agency. The agency advertised for accounting positions and for office jobs. I knew I did not want to work in retail. I either wanted to work outside or in an office, but no retail. The temp agency advertised that they specialized in accounting and office work, which was definitely not retail. The ad suggested a phone call, or I could email my résumé in. I emailed my résumé, and the agency called me within an hour. I had an appointment the next Monday to interview and to take some accounting skills assessment tests. Laura and I rushed to the library, and I boned up on my accounting skills with a few borrowed books.

On that Monday morning, I took the tests, scored extremely high, and interviewed with one of the agents. She told me she would have me placed in a few weeks. I arrived home that afternoon feeling great. Finally, there was some movement on the job front. Rather unexpectedly, that same day around 4 P.M., I received a call from the agent. Did I want to start work tomorrow?

She described the company and the job. It was a temp job filling in for someone on maternity leave. It paid $9.50 an hour, a third of what I'd been making in Arizona, but a heckuva a lot more per hour than $0. I said yes. When I told Laura, we both cried in relief. I was at work the next day by 9:00 A.M. and at my desk by 9:15 A.M. I was there to support two sales directors who were responsible for a couple hundred million dollars in revenue. That sum seemed so large that it was more like play money than real cash. By the end of the first day, most of the people I was working with were asking me what my story was and why was I working as a temp at $9.50 an hour.

I shared with them the cancer story. By the end of the second day, the two sales directors wanted to know if I wanted a full-time job. They would want me to guarantee I would support them and their teams for a year. After the year, we would evaluate where I was professionally and what I would want to do. They offered me $32,500 a year with full benefits and a potential bonus. I said Yes.

A year later, I had kept my word, and they did as well. I moved into a full-time sales role and ended up as a sales director there before moving on. The day I received my first job post-cancer, Laura and I had 79 cents left in our bank account. I received my first paycheck that Friday. The company I worked for got me a $1,000 signing bonus as soon as I agreed to a full-time job. One of the directors gave the check to me and said simply, "We know you need this." My friend, God provides. And He was not finished providing and blessing us.

What does the word "providence" mean to you?

How have you seen God provide for you in your life?

Who have you told about His provision?

Luke 12:24 (ESV): "Consider the ravens: they neither sow nor reap, they have neither storehouse nor barn, and yet God feeds them. Of how much more value are you than the birds!"

2 Corinthians 5:17 (ESV): "Therefore, if anyone is in Christ, he is a new creation.

Chapter 30

By late 2004, life was getting back to what I considered normal. I was back on health insurance. I was seeing doctors who continued the great care I had received in Arizona, and I had a career again. My new oncology doctors at IU were virtually the same as my oncology team out in Arizona. I cannot recommend IU as a medical provider enough. My oncologist in Indiana had been advising my oncologist in Arizona. I was able to meet and be under the care of the doctor who developed the protocol to cure my cancer. The team at IU is an amazing and caring group of top-notch physicians.

And something else happened. God was not through with His provision.

Laura and I became pregnant.

Laura and I started trying to have our second child around the time I took on the full-time sales role. It did not take long before Laura shared the awesome news that she was pregnant. All of my doctors, all of them, insisted there was no way Laura and I could have a baby together naturally. I believed them; Laura did not. When we started trying to get pregnant, I did not expect anything to happen. So it was a great surprise to me personally when Laura's pregnancy test came back positive.

We both cried a great deal, rejoiced even more, and prayed, and prayed, and prayed. We did not tell anyone for a few months, as we wanted to make sure our baby was healthy and that there were no complications. The pregnancy went well, except that Laura had severe nausea and incredibly strong acid indigestion for the entire pregnancy.

I was pretty much in shock, but I should not have been. God had been so faithful and Laura so strong that I should have foreseen that they would team up on this one. The pregnancy went very well and incredibly fast. The day approached quicker than I could have imagined. We, of course, had people praying again, all over the world. We were having a daughter this time, and the idea of me having a daughter was terrifying.

In early October, Laura went into labor, just after our son's fourth birthday. Laura's parents were staying with us at the time. All of us had spent that day together, walking around downtown Indy, hitting as many monuments as we could. Walking always seemed to move things along for Laura. It did this time as well. Her water broke that night, and we headed to the hospital.

Laura's first labor had gone OK, but I needed help, so we hired a doula for our second child. Our doula became a very good friend of ours. A doula, according to Google's dictionary, is a woman, typically without formal obstetric training, who is employed to provide guidance and support to a pregnant woman during labor. I always thought of our doula as a labor coach helping Laura, and me, during the delivery. We were still living near downtown Indy, so our delivery was at one of the major downtown hospitals. When Laura went into labor, we were out of the house and into the hospital within 15 minutes.

The delivery went very quickly. Laura was in good shape. The baby's vital signs all showed positive, no distress, everything seemed great. I was praying, of course, and for some dumb reason, I got the idea in my head that this baby would be mine. We had given our son to God; he was our firstborn, and we had dedicated him to the Lord. I just kept thinking and praying about how this one would be mine.

When our baby girl came out, I could tell something was wrong immediately. She was not moving and she was an odd color. The cord had wrapped itself around her neck, and had choked her on the way out. She was not breathing. Her skin was blue, especially her lips. The medical staff looked at her, looked at each other, and then called in the Neonatal Intensive Care Unit (NICU).

Our doula caught my eye and visibly shared a great deal of concern. I panicked inside, and then Laura asked what was wrong. I looked at Laura and at our doula, took a deep breath, and said, "She will be fine." There was no sign of life, and I begged God for her to survive. I asked God to forgive my selfishness, and that this daughter, and any other children we might have, would be entirely dedicated to Him. I would be a caretaker and lead them, but ultimately, every child would be His.

The NICU people were in that room with all of their equipment in less than a minute. They took our daughter, unwrapped and cut the cord, and then they placed her in a warming unit and very carefully resuscitated her. Laura and I stood there holding hands. My wife was crying, and so was I.

We watched these amazing people work to save the life of our daughter. And what felt like an eternity later, they announced she was breathing. Her temperature was rising. Her limbs were moving. The NICU nurse pulled me aside and said our daughter was not out of danger yet, and they would not know her full condition until later. They were going to take her into the NICU critical care area, and I would be allowed to go back to see her. My wife would not be allowed to see her at first, as there were some post-birth items to take care of.

A few minutes passed as Laura and the medical staff finished up what needed to be completed to take care of Laura. Eventually a nurse came and tugged on my arm. None of us had received any further word, and I was led back to the critical care area. Our daughter was in a crib with an oxygen hood covering her. She was lying on her stomach. Her color was good. Her skin tone is a darker hue like mine, so she was not pink, but she was not pasty white or blue, either.

The nurse monitoring her spoke to me quietly and said I could not touch her yet, but I could speak to her. The nurse asked me her name, which I could not answer as Laura and I had not named her yet. We had been debating over her name for months, so when the nurse asked me her name, I told her quietly that we were debating between two names. Our daughter had a mass of thick, black curly hair. Her face was turned away from me. Without thinking, instinctively, I called her by one of the names we had chosen. I said something like, "Hey, look at you!" Much to the nurse's amazement, and my own, this newborn baby girl stirred. I said her name again. This little newborn girl then did a full pushup and turned her head to look at me. We were face to face for the first time. This beautiful baby girl with brown eyes that matched my own was staring into me. My heart broke, and my life has never been the same again. I was totally helpless, lost, proud, and madly in love all over again. This little girl continued to stare at me as I babbled and cried all over her.

The nurse put her hand on my shoulder and said, "She is going to be fine. I have never seen a newborn complete a full pushup like that, let alone turn her head. She'll be fine." I was ushered out again, as they needed to further test her, which she passed with flying colors. I went back into the room with my wife and our doula, who were waiting expectantly for me and any news. They both looked very worried. I was stunned at how this little girl had so drastically changed me as a father and a man. I would never look at women the same way again. When I walked into the room, I was glowing.

The news about our daughter was all over the ward, and nurses came in to make sure my wife knew our daughter was fine. I told Laura and our doula what had happened, and all three of us sobbed and prayed. While we were huddled together, our daughter was brought in, and Laura got to hold her for the first time.

We had a few hiccups over the next 30 days, mainly due to our daughter developing a urinary tract infection. However, her heart and her brain functioned incredibly well. Our insurance at the time was decent, but we did owe quite a bit of money for the birth and the NICU work. As we typically do, we decided to set up payments for our medical bills. When Laura called to set up payments a month or two later, the business manager told us our debt to the hospital was forgiven. And that is how she put it: our debt was forgiven. The medical staff had gathered together, prayed, and felt led to forgive whatever we owed the hospital. Our daughter is living proof of God's provision and His faithfulness to us. And God was not through. We have had two more children after our daughter—three children our medical team said were impossible—another son and then another daughter. With God all things are possible. We cherish all four, and each has been given over and dedicated to the Lord. Without Him, we would not have had other children. How could we do anything less?

Life has not been all bells and whistles. We still have our struggles. I have fought a severe case of diverticulitis. I had three holes in my intestinal tract that took me months to recover from, and none of it was pleasant. We struggled with job loss, financial need, illness, and deaths in our family.

In between the birth of our youngest son and our youngest daughter, both of whom broke my heart and caused me to fall in love all over again, we became pregnant with our baby number four, chronologically. Our youngest daughter is actually our fifth pregnancy. Unfortunately, our fourth child did not survive. On September 17, 2009, the baby we named Riley passed on. Many of our friends and our family would say we lost the baby. The baby is not lost. We know exactly where and with whom Riley is, and one day Laura and I will get to meet her in heaven. As Jesus tells us in Matthew 19:14b (ESV), "For of [children] is the kingdom of heaven."

I firmly believe our child along with millions and millions of other children fill heaven. For those of us who are believers, and whose young children have gone on ahead, by one way or another, we will see those children again, or as in our case, for the first time.

Our joy is in the Lord. He has been faithful and has blessed us beyond measure. The suffering, the doubt, and the fear we experienced all led us to a place where we know God is who He said He is, and He is to be trusted. Suffering can lead to joy, regardless of circumstance when we trust Him.

Has God surprised you with a child? Natural, adoptive, or foster?

How did the child change your view of life, of the world?

Has God ever told you No? How are your trusting Him through the No?

Psalm 127 (ESV): "Unless the Lord builds the house, those who build it labor in vain. Unless the Lord watches over the city, the watchman stays awake in vain. It is in vain that you rise up early and go late to rest, eating the bread of anxious toil; for he gives to his beloved sleep.

"Behold, children are a heritage from the Lord, the fruit of the womb a reward. Like arrows in the hand of a warrior are the children of one's youth. Blessed is the man who fills his quiver with them! He shall not be put to shame when he speaks with his enemies in the gate."

Epilogue

If you have made it this far, bear with me for a little while longer. My assumption is you are reading this book because you are either fighting cancer yourself, or you have a loved one who is fighting cancer, or you are suffering in some way. It is also possible someone you know who cares for you knows of your struggles has put this book in your hands. My hope and prayer is that this story of my own battle with cancer and God's ever-present provision has been one of encouragement.

By now, it should be quite obvious that I am a follower of Christ Jesus. I came to a saving knowledge and a trust of Him before my cancer battle began. My anchor through the entire ordeal was Him and His Word. I would be dishonest in telling my story without His involvement in it, and I would be in error if I did not extend to you the opportunity to know Him.

Whether you are fighting cancer, or you are fighting cancer alongside a loved one, or are in another dire struggle, you have a much bigger problem. All of us do. We live in a universe created by a holy God, a God who loves us but who is so separate, so different from us that He is hard for us to fathom. This Creator is perfect. He is without sin, and because of His Holiness, He is unable to accept us unless we are also without blemish. He cannot accept those who do not accept Him. To do so would be a kind of theft. Because He is a loving God, we also have an opportunity, all of us do.

God is well aware of how we are in our hearts, our errors, our foibles, and our sin. We get angry and we hate. You don't believe me? Try watching the news for more than five minutes on the news channel you never watch. Try it—the odds are it will make you angry. We get angry enough in our hearts to hurt or kill, even though we may never carry it out.

We cuss; we take His name in vain. We steal (how many pens do you have at home from work?). We cheat. Have you ever looked at someone who is not your spouse and desired him or her? Did you desire that person enough to think about what it would be like? That's adultery in your heart.

Have you ever lied? Ever?

I have struggled with all of these sins in my life. All of them. I am no different than anyone else.

The sad truth is, it only takes one sin to separate us from God. Can you honestly say you have never committed a single sin? Never? I cannot.

So where is the opportunity, where is the hope when confronted with the simple truth that we all fall short of God's expectations?

The opportunity is provided to us by God Himself. He knows our shortcomings. He knows our sin. And shockingly, He loves us despite our sin, despite our opposition to Him. We live in a culture in which performance is always king. In God's economy, His love is not conditioned on our performance. Instead, because of His love, He made a way for us—a way to Him for eternity. It is a way we have to choose for ourselves. No one else can make this choice. We have to freely choose Him.

The Apostle Paul tells us in 1 Timothy 2:4 (ESV) that our desire for God, "who desires all people to be saved and to come to the knowledge of the truth," is a conditional desire. We have to make the choice. And the choice we need to make is Jesus Christ.

Do we accept Him as Savior, or do we dismiss Him? According to scripture, Jesus lived a sinless life and then paid for our sins on the Cross at Calvary. In rising on the third day, He proved He is who He said He was, and He has the power to save us. And by dying a substitutionary death for our sin, being buried, and rising again, this amazing, loving, holy God made a way for us to be with Him for all eternity. The way is through His Son.

Romans 10:9–13 (ESV): "Because, if you confess with your mouth that Jesus is Lord and believe in your heart that God raised him from the dead, you will be saved. For with the heart one believes and is justified, and with the mouth one confesses and is saved. For the Scripture says, 'Everyone who believes in him will not be put to shame.' For there is no distinction between Jew and Greek; for the same Lord is Lord of all, bestowing his riches on all who call on him. For 'everyone who calls on the name of the Lord will be saved.'"

I believe that not only will Christ Jesus save all who have turned to Him, confessed their sin to Him, and believe He is Lord, I also believe that Jesus won't leave them be. He will also begin to work inside them, through the Holy Spirit, and while painful at times, the life we can have here and now, no matter how short that life might be, is vastly superior than anything we could possibly imagine without Him.

I also believe that Jesus has the power to heal us. He healed me physically, spiritually, and emotionally. He allowed me to forgive people who wounded me so grievously that their actions adversely affected me for decades. And in forgiving them, I was able to free myself.

My friend, I do not know if Jesus will heal you physically or not. I know He can. God can do anything. He did completely heal me. I do not know if he will heal you. He may or He may not. Regardless of whether He does heal you or not, I will, as all Christians should,

"Rejoice with you when you rejoice, and weep with you when you weep" (Romans 12:15). You are not alone.

I may have cancer again some day. I have had it twice in my life, after all. Mind you, I hope I never have cancer again. However, if I do, I know where I am going when I pass on. As the apostle Paul said in Romans 8:18, "For I consider that the sufferings of this present time are not worth comparing with the glory that is to be revealed to us." What we have in the future with Him is so much grander and glorious than what we suffer through this day, for today is not even comparable to our future with Him.

Beloved, Jesus wants you to be His, now and forever. He wants you to know that you are not alone. He wants you as you are, wherever you are, whatever you are going through.

Have you accepted Christ? Do you believe in Him? Will you be saved?

I invite you to accept Him. Won't you accept Him today? Now? Please say yes to Him.

To my fellow believers, to my brothers and sisters in Christ, I hope you have found encouragement as well. I struggled for years about the Why of it all. Why is a question we like to ask often. Why is this happening to me? Why Lord? Why?

"Why" is an absolutely fair question. And "why" is a question God does not always answer, at least not directly. What I can share with you, if you are asking Why and you are a believer, is this: You trust God for your eternal destiny, your eternal salvation. And you are right to do so.

You can also trust Him in this. You can trust Him in cancer. You can trust Him in job loss. You can trust Him in suffering, in His silence, in your circumstance. If you can trust Christ for your life after this one, you can and should trust Him with this life, as well. Be unshakable. He is the rock; lean on Him, lean on His promise to us.

We may be fighting cancer. We may be suffering. However, we are His. We are no longer victims. We are conquerors. As Paul reminds us in **Romans 8:37–39** (ESV): "No, in all these things we are more than conquerors through Him who loved us. For I am sure that neither death nor life, nor angels nor rulers, nor things present nor things to come, nor powers, nor height nor depth, nor anything else in all creation, will be able to separate us from the love of God in Christ Jesus our Lord."

Will you trust Him even in this, your struggle?

I pray nightly for those who are fighting cancer, who are suffering. I pray for strength, for wisdom, and for salvation. May God deliver you, and help you to find peace in Him. God bless!

CPSIA information can be obtained
at www.ICGtesting.com
Printed in the USA
LVHW040626121020
668550LV00004B/309